INTOXICATING LIES

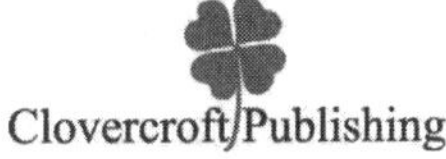

Intoxicating Lies: One Woman's Journey to Freedom from Gray Area Drinking

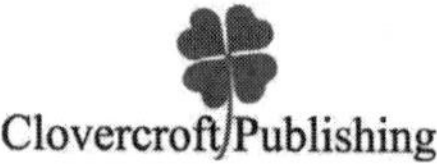

Published by Clovercroft Publishing, Franklin, Tennessee
Published in association with Shane Crabtree of Clovercroft Publishing
www.clovercroftpublishing.com

Cover and Interior Design by Melinda Martin
Edited by Gail Fallen
Author Photo by Robbyn Dodd Photography

Printed in the United States of America

ISBN: 978-1-954437-63-0 (paperback)

Meg Geisewite
Foreword by Jenn Kautsch

INTOXICATING LIES

ONE WOMAN'S JOURNEY TO FREEDOM FROM GRAY AREA DRINKING

Clovercroft Publishing

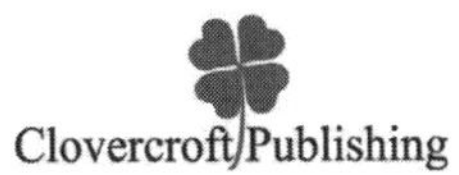

To my husband, Paul, you are my North Star.
We cannot control the winds and storms of life,
but your steadfast, radical acceptance of me
on this journey has been a guiding light.

For your unconditional love and encouragement,
I am forever grateful.

CONTENTS

Preface.........vii

Foreword.........ix

INTRODUCTION The Little Engine That Could.........1

CHAPTER ONE "I Deserve a Glass".........3

CHAPTER TWO "You Don't Have a Drinking Problem"20

CHAPTER THREE "I Can Control My Drinking".........45

CHAPTER FOUR "Being Sober Is Boring".........63

CHAPTER FIVE "Behind Every Great Mom Is a Bottle of Wine".........89

CHAPTER SIX "Go Ahead, You Can Have a Sip".........103

CHAPTER SEVEN The End of the Merry-Go-Round.........117

CHAPTER EIGHT The Truth of Who You Are.........133

Conclusion.........145

Note from the Author.........147

Tools to Explore Your Alcohol-Free Journey.........149

Early Entries from My Alcohol-Free Journal.........157

Acknowledgments.........159

About the Author.........163

Endnotes.........165

FOREWORD

I believe everything happens for a reason and individual journeys connect together along an invisible timeline when both people are ready to intersect.

It was time for our paths to cross when Meg participated in my 21-Day Reset Challenge in Fall 2019. As founder of the Sober Sis Tribe, I'm honored to be a part of her story and have her as a pillar in our community of SoberMinded Sisters. We connected as two women on the same trail aiming to reach the heights of becoming the best version of ourselves. I've been her guide along the way, just a few steps ahead.

Often, when women come into Sober Sis, I have no idea the backstory and how many steps have already been taken to get to this place of openness, readiness, and curiosity. In an alcohol-centric world, it's very brave to pull over from the drinking highway and "pop the hood" in one's life to see what's really going on.

Meg has a way of taking the truths she's learned and breathing in a fresh perspective through her personal experience. Her stories are so relatable and inspire other women to understand they are *not* alone.

Meg is the "real deal" because she is truly living a life of freedom. She is fully awakening to the inner healing and resilience that was buried inside because of the lies around alcohol . . . that ultimately led to the lies she believed about herself.

Through the past few years of coaching, I've seen many women change and transform their lives. I've just seen a handful who can articulate at this level and allow the reader to feel as if they are embarking on a personal journey too!

I know you will enjoy reading *Intoxicating Lies* as much as I have! The goal is to encourage open conversation and extend an invitation to see alcohol differently . . . exposing the intoxicating lies that the marketing and messaging whispers (or screams) to us women every day. Knowledge is power, and when we know better, we can *choose* better.

Cheers!

Jenn Kautsch
Founder/CEO, Sober Sis
Sobersis.com/ss-home

PREFACE

Everyone wants to feel like they have control in their life. We want to believe that we always have a choice. We especially want to believe that the things we started doing for pleasure or for fun are still just that—pleasurable and fun. Because everyone else is doing it too.

But for many of us, alcohol slowly starts to turn on us, leaving an unsettled feeling deep inside. Your desire to let loose a little or unwind has turned into a nightly habit of filing down the rough edges of your day. You start to wake up in the middle of the night or in the morning feeling this isn't that fun anymore. You start to wonder if this is causing you harm.

So maybe you find yourself questioning your relationship with alcohol. Maybe you find yourself cleansing from alcohol for a thirty-day challenge like "Sober September" or "Dry January" only to slip back into your old drinking ways shortly thereafter. Maybe you tell yourself, *After the holidays or this upcoming wedding, I will cut back* or *I won't drink during the week—only on the weekends*, but you fall short in following your own rules.

I felt just like you. I felt alone, confused, and crazy. Everyone around me was drinking on par with me, yet I felt trapped in a toxic relationship with alcohol. I felt guilt for not being able to control my relationship with alcohol and shame for my behavior. If you know how this feels, let me assure you: You are *not* crazy, and you are *not* alone. You may have fallen into the same trap so many people are held hostage in today called "gray area drinking."

I always thought you were either a "normal" drinker or a "problematic, rock-bottom" drinker. I did not realize there was an alcohol use disorder spectrum, let alone a category called gray area drinking. I did not relate to the rock-bottom drinking stories, and that kept me trapped in an addiction of gray area drinking for many years, not realizing that I needed help. Everyone was safe—there weren't any negative external consequences. My job was not in the throes of disaster because of my drinking. I never got behind the wheel after drinking. I wasn't being reckless or indulging in risky behavior. I never drank during the day, though I did drink most evenings.

Even though my behavior looked safe and normal on the outside, I couldn't escape the nagging feeling that something was wrong. I felt trapped and fearful of expressing my concern about my drinking pattern. I was on a continuous loop of waking up feeling like crap. Working off my slight hangover all day at work, managing the kids and my home productively, all while convincing myself that I was in control of my relationship with alcohol. My late afternoon workouts furthered my belief that I was handling it.

I was a divided woman with a divided heart. The daylight hours were my "convincing hours," constantly reassuring myself that I still had a choice . . . that was, until the sun set. Right around dinnertime, my brain would start to flip its script, telling me that I not only needed alcohol but that I also *deserved* it. Everyone's needs were taken care of that day but mine. My all-day mantra of "I won't drink tonight" slowly transformed into a new voice within my head: *Go ahead, it's only one glass. You biked twenty miles today, you don't have a problem. You deserve to relax, unwind with a glass of wine. All your friends have their nightly wine and don't have a problem.* And so on.

I allowed my cravings to wash over me in the evenings, succumbing to a glass of wine that was *never* just one glass. The next morning, I'd wake with shame and regret, wondering why I couldn't get this under control.

What I have learned since then is that the alcohol industry and our society want to keep you small, quiet, and thinking you are the problem. Like Valium in the 1960s, alcohol has become the new "Mommy's Little Helper," targeting women who truly do need support and offering them a new mode of "self-care." And, like Valium, alcohol *works*. It's easily accessible, socially acceptable, and widely praised in the media. Everyone is invested in keeping up the illusion that alcohol is fun, harmless, and—most importantly for women—*deserved*. Acknowledging you have questions or doubts about it makes you the odd woman out.

The fear and stigma associated with facing these questions keep us addicted and silent. Gray area drinking is a surprisingly common problem on the alcohol use disorder spectrum that we are not talking about enough. There are so many people, particularly women, trapped in this cyclical hell of a detoxing only to "retox" again because we are hooked on this highly celebrated, highly addictive drug.

I want you to know you are not alone in this quest to understand why you cannot control your relationship with alcohol. I wanted to explore my relationship with alcohol and decided to do a private online 21-Day Reset Challenge with Sober Sis, a community of (at the time) over five thousand sober-curious women, to get my drinking back in shape. I figured it was my issue—that I just needed to reign it in a bit. I was not ready to break up with alcohol.

When I joined Sober Sis, I was floored that so many women felt like I did. I was not alone by far. (As I write this, there are now over twenty-five thousand women in Sober Sis who have participated in the 21-Day Reset Challenge and thousands who have gone on to living an alcohol-free life.) My intuition wasn't wrong. During my journey, it became apparent that alcohol had played a big role in dimming and doubting my inner knowing. Slowly, I started to realign with my inner knowing—your intrinsic wisdom otherwise known as your intuition.

If you are sick and tired of being sick and tired from alcohol, you have come to the right place. If you are unsure whether you can reclaim your life, *you can*. You are not alone. If the merry-go-round and tug of war in your head with alcohol is making you feel crazy, trust your inner knowing and keep reading.

In this book, I will take you through my journey of uncovering the intoxicating lies of alcohol and introduce you to many other women who are just like you. Each chapter outlines the lies about alcohol I told myself over and over again for years and reveals the truth that we need to know. We will learn about the gray area drinking spectrum, how we fall into the alcohol trap, and how to navigate your way out of unhealthy habits, roles, and expectations from our culture to wholehearted living and reconnecting to yourself.

You will also hear from other women in my Sober Sis group whose stories are different from mine but who shared the same underlying thread of being seduced by the lies of alcohol and the benefits we believed it provided to our lives. The names of these women have been changed to protect their identities. I hope that our journeys support you on your own unique path to reconnect to your inner knowing, your true self, by exposing the intoxicating lies of alcohol.

Finally, I am not an expert, a doctor, or a treatment specialist. I am a mother who felt trapped by gray area drinking for years and who was looking for a book that met me where I was, and I could not find anything on the market at that time. I do not have all the answers, but I hope this book opens your eyes to the truths about alcohol. This book is not designed to diagnose or treat anyone but rather increase the conversation about this rarely discussed gray area drinking space on the alcohol use disorder spectrum. This is not a book on how to get sober. It is an exploration of an alcohol-free journey.

My hope is that this book makes you more curious about the illusions and lies created by the alcohol industry and our alcohol-centric society. By the end of this book, I hope my journey leaves you feeling empowered by dismantling and debunking these myths about alcohol and the damaging messages we get from society. I hope you will feel liberated and free from the confusion and ingrained messages, especially to women, regarding alcohol and your worth. I applaud you for taking the next step to exploring your relationship with alcohol.

Now it's time to get curious!

INTRODUCTION

THE LITTLE ENGINE THAT COULD

You might know the classic children's book (or film) *The Little Engine That Could*. When I was growing up, my dad would always say to me, "You are my little engine that could." This stuck with me even into my adult years: I was always striving, pushing, never stopping, always going after the perfect partner, the perfect job, the perfect house, the perfect body, and so on. Always needing to be in control, my little engine would work harder and harder every day to make sure it looked like I had it all. It was a shiny cable car, chugging up hills and gliding around turns, making it all look easy when in reality, it was not. *I think I can—I think I can—I think I can. . . .*

My little engine was exhausted. I needed a place to rest and found solace in alcohol. Then, when major life events happened all at once and I could not control them, I started making daily stops to refuel with alcohol at a "drinking station" to let off some steam. I didn't know how to handle all the feelings that surged upon me, but at 5 p.m., after running and pushing my engine over mountains all day, I finally shut off my engine and consoled myself with a drink. Over time, alcohol became synonymous with my self-care, like a lubricant on my engine, making me believe it ran better with a drink.

The irony of my drinking was that it started as a place to relinquish control, but in actuality it took control of *me*. My little engine went in circles for years, chugging harder and harder to the tune of "I Think I Can," trying to regain control. What I didn't realize at the time was that I had a one-way ticket back to the same refueling station, day in and day out. I knew it in my heart, but everyone around me looked like their shiny engines were functioning just as well as mine, so I continued on the route to nowhere. In the children's book, the little engine's main job was to provide for all the little boys and girls, much like women often have to provide, nurture, and mother all the people in our lives. Little did I realize at the time, I was falling further and further into gray area drinking. My engine was exhausted, sick, and needed help.

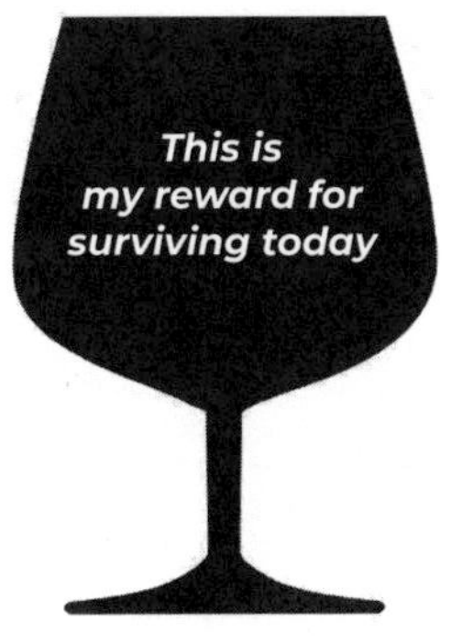

CHAPTER ONE

"I DESERVE A GLASS"

On November 1, 2019, I woke up to one of the worst hangovers I had had in a long time. My head throbbed as I slowly climbed out of bed to get dressed for work. Fog and grayness were my lens through which I saw the world that day and, quite frankly, most of my days. My stomach gurgled, sending me running to the bathroom every fifteen minutes to try to get some relief from the knots of nausea that entangled my gut. Once again, I had to pull it off at my pharmaceutical sales job like nothing had happened the night before. I was meeting my medical science liaison for breakfast and was about to take a deep dive into new research that had come out on my product. I got to the restaurant early, grabbing a large coffee and a biscuit to line my stomach. My hands trembled from the bottomless prosecco the night before. I tried to clear out the fogginess in my mind to stay astute as my colleague teased apart all the new data to help me sell my therapy to physicians.

Knowing that today would be the first day of my 21-Day Sober Sis Reset Challenge, I had overindulged the night before, on Halloween. I was trick-or-treating with some friends, excited to have an excuse to drink more than my usual couple of glasses of wine at night. It was a crisp fall evening, and all of us were dressed in costume, pretending we were something we were not. We had our large Yeti cups filled to the brim with prosecco. As we meandered throughout my friend's neighborhood, the treat in my Yeti was dwindling fast. I was concerned I would run out of my drink before the kids were done gathering candy. My treat, alcohol, had tricked me and was in complete control of my thoughts. This was normal for me. Alcohol dictated my mood, signaling the end of my day, ringing with persistent urgency to get my drink on to unwind. It became a priority for me over everything else at the end of the day.

Getting low on our prosecco, we decided to head back to my girlfriend's house for refills. One of the girls in the trick-or-treating group asked me quietly, "Do you drink every night?"

My thoughts raced. Do I tell her the truth or lie? She was drinking on pace with me, so I thought, *What the hell, I'll tell her the truth.*

"Yes, yes, I do," I replied with an embarrassed chuckle.

She replied, "Whew, me too."

As she was a prominent, successful lawyer (and a businesswoman like me), we both found commonality and condolence in our gray area of drinking.

My girlfriend continued with her questioning: "How much do you drink?"

We had already gotten this far, so I replied again truthfully, "Sometimes a couple glasses of wine a night, but many times it is the entire bottle, which is only really three big glasses of wine, if we are being honest."

"Oh, thank God, me too!" she exclaimed. In some odd way, it was good to know I was not alone, but it was also frightening to wonder: We both looked like we had our shit together, but did we *really*?

After the trick-or-treating was over, I took an Uber home with my son, because I never drank and drove. I always felt good about my choice to not drink and drive, as if that in itself was proof that I was fine. But when I got home, I continued to drink. I knew I had a problem. I knew it was in control of me. When I no longer wanted my kids to do sports in the evenings so I could come home after work to my rewarding wine, I knew I had lost myself in the bottle. I had known it for some time.

Where It All Started

Growing up as the oldest sibling of three, I was the rule follower, the caretaker, and the overachiever in my family. I was the good girl who never wanted to disappoint my parents. The house I lived in the longest was in one of the wealthiest zip codes in Delaware. Large, lush green oak trees lined the streets of the perfectly manicured estates, sheltering the homes from the reality of the world. Our circle was small; everyone knew everyone. Most of my days were spent at the country club, where I was on the swim team, took tennis lessons, and learned ballroom dancing to attend cotillion. Each week, my brother, sister, and I would dress up in our best attire to learn the foxtrot, waltz, or the cha-cha-cha in the grand ballroom.

Weekends included evening country-club cocktail parties for the adults, where the alcohol flowed freely. Whenever my parents hosted, my mom would dress me up in my best Jessica McClintock velvet dress and I would serve hors d'oeuvres to our inebriated guests, all while smiling and learning how to people please at a very early age. Unbeknownst to me (and through no fault of my parents, who were also conditioned with this old, programmed belief), the messages that alcohol was a way to connect with others coupled with concern for how we appeared to others were both slowly being ingrained into my subconscious.

My dad's job moved us frequently throughout my childhood. We lived in nine houses in four states. I can clearly remember being in yet another new private school, with no friends, going up to girls who I barely knew, asking, "Hi, my name is Meg. Do you want to be friends and come to my birthday party?" My birthday is the first week of September, when school begins, so there was little time to develop friendships before my birthday. Learning how to make friends quickly served me well in all our travels. Being friendly, outgoing, and people pleasing were traits I was honing from the first grade.

In the fifth grade, my parents took all three of us—my brother, sister, and me—to a prominent psychiatrist to have our IQs tested. Back then, aptitude testing was normal, especially in the circle my parents ran in. This psychiatrist was well respected within our community. She was a frequent guest at our Christmas parties, and it was a given that her services would be rendered when we were the right age. I sat down in her office staring up at her academic accolades on her wall. She handed me a pencil and a bunch of papers stapled together. I was annoyed that I would be stuck in her office for a few hours completing a battery of tests.

When I finished all the questions, she studied me with her big black round glasses and inquisitive eyes. As her large ornate silver necklace dangled in front of my face, she asked me to draw a picture. I loved drawing and had taken several art classes outside of school.

As I drew the picture, she was totaling up my score from the IQ test. Upon completion of my drawing, she picked up my artwork and said in so many words, "Your score was low . . . it's a good thing you can draw because you don't have much else going for you."

All I heard was "You won't amount to much." Since she was the expert, and I was a naïve little girl, I kept her hurtful, damaging words to myself.

That same year, at my all-girls Catholic middle school, I was ostracized by my circle of friends. Now the message of "You don't belong here" was swirling and spiraling in my head, along with "You'll never amount to much." I cried almost every day when I got home from school. The pain of not having any friends and getting glaring stares from the popular group in class forced me into the nurse's office almost daily to escape the pain. After a year of this turmoil, my mom pulled me out of that school and put me into public school. Now the need to fit in was of utmost importance to me.

Like I always did at new schools, I made new friends quickly. In eighth grade, I had my first sleepover with the popular girls, where we raided my parents' liquor cabinet. I desperately wanted to fit in, to be part of the popular group, so I thought a few shots of peach schnapps would seal the deal. I felt I earned points with the popular girls that night at my slumber party, but I spent the entire next day throwing up.

My very first hangover.

Even as awful as that first hangover was, I felt early on that drinking gave me the attention I wanted and needed to fit in during high school. My mom used to always say to me when I got caught drinking in high school, "You punish yourself by drinking that much," which was true, but it did not stop me. There was never an explanation as to why I was punishing myself. There were no messages about the dangers of drinking in high school other than "Don't drink and drive" and "Don't drink if you are pregnant." That was about it.

Tragically, I learned the lesson about drinking and driving the hard way my freshman year of high school. I was not allowed to go to parties. It was Saturday night; I had been at a sleepover the night before with a few friends. I lay in bed thinking of a fib to tell my parents so that I could go to this big party that my entire high school had been talking about all week. I fell asleep, wiped out from staying up all night the night before.

I awoke the next morning to the gut-wrenching news that my friends had been in a horrific drinking and driving accident. The party had gotten so big and out of control that the police raided the party, leaving my friends to jump into a car with someone who was drunk to escape getting caught by the police. Hearing the story, the bottom of my stomach dropped out: I realized if I had not fallen asleep while trying to think of a lie to go to the party, I would have been in that car with my friends.

Tragically, I lost one of my best friends in that godforsaken accident. I was forever changed. I became president of our high school's SADD (now known as Students Against Destructive Decisions) chapter. I vowed never to drink and drive in honor of Carla's life—a life which was taken too quickly and senselessly. It's a vow I have kept to this day.

During this impressionable time, I got into modeling. My parents enrolled me into a modeling school and my dad even took me to New York City to some of the big modeling agencies. Even though I did not land a big contract, I did several modeling gigs over the course of a few years to earn money. It was here that I started gaining praise for my appearance. Modeling school further ingrained how to appear to the outside world: how to have proper etiquette, how to carry myself, how to look and act the part of perfectionism and people pleasing.

Back then, my idols were supermodels (like Cindy Crawford and Christy Turlington, who ruled the runways). This insatiable quest for the unattainable look illustrated in magazines and on television only reinforced what I believed being truly "beautiful" meant. I started looking outside of myself more than ever, allowing the world to validate my worth and slowly disconnect from myself.

Perfectionism, coupled with a need to fit in and prove that I was enough, led to a high-school career of sacrificing what I loved to do, which was ice skating, so I could cheerlead and be with the popular girls once again. I even joined the band (yes, band was cool in my high school; in fact, it was a rite of passage to *being* cool) even though I could not read music. The band director put me on the cymbals, and the drum major would nod my way when it was time to clang the cymbals. It's funny looking back, but it's also sad seeing my desperation to fit in. I continued to drink in high school, only at parties where I could sneak a few in to be part of the gang. I drank just like my friends on occasions where it was never a problem. Unknowingly, the subliminal messages of "This is how you have a good time and fit in" were being further etched into my brain.

Little did I know that during these formative years when you are trying to find yourself, your people, and where you fit into this big world, my world was about to be turned upside down. During my junior year of high school, my parents sat me, my brother, and my sister down for a talk at dinner one night. They looked at each other and said, "We have decided to take a 'time-out'; we don't even want to call it a separation."

Stunned, my siblings and I just sat at the dinner table in silence, staring at each other in bewilderment. It was confusing for us as we barely saw our parents fight, but behind closed doors it was a different story. They could not agree on much and once apart (officially separated), it became vividly clear how different they really were. It wasn't long after their time-out that they decided to divorce. Our family unit was crumbling; pieces were falling so fast around me that I didn't know how the puzzle would ever come back together.

I come from a big Italian family on my mom's side, where getting together and being together took precedence over pretty much anything else. We constantly had family parties, celebrations, and get-togethers for any and every reason. Our biggest and most cherished get-together was the annual Christmas party at my aunt and uncle's mansion. My twenty-three cousins and I would run around playing games, getting lost in each of the massive home's wings and multiple staircases.

I was running through the kitchen when my aunt stopped me and pulled me into her butler's pantry. Alone, just the two of us, she said to me with tears in her eyes, "Meg, I am so sorry about your parent's divorce. You are the oldest and you will have to take care of your brother and sister through all of this." I remember thinking *I was just playing hide-and-go-seek with my little cousins*, and now the enormity of my parents' divorce and how it would play out for us was laid squarely on my shoulders.

"This will not be easy," she continued, "and you will need to be there for your brother and sister."

I just nodded like a good girl, knowing that being the oldest had its fair share of responsibilities and now this one was going to be one of the bigger ones on my plate. I swallowed the lump in my throat, pushing aside my feelings and needs, knowing that my role of caretaker had just grown exponentially.

An Education in Shame

It was now time for me to go off to college, leaving my brother and sister to fend for themselves through our parents' messy divorce. As we toured college campuses, my parents would ask the college tour guide about their rape statistics. No matter which college we were considering, my mom always told me, "If anything happens to you, you can just come home and go to University of Delaware." That was the *last* place I wanted to be—with all my high school friends. I needed a new chapter, new friends: I needed out of our small state. The zero degrees of separation in little ole Delaware had taken a toll on me.

I settled on a college six hours from home, far enough away from the turmoil of the divorce. Even though there were hundreds of miles between me and my past, the words "You'll never amount to much" still rang through my head as I raced from extracurricular activity to extracurricular activity on campus to prove my worth. Alcohol, particularly beer, was more readily available in college where two dollars got you into any keg party on campus.

One night, I was imbibing at one of these on-campus keg parties when a good-looking, muscular rugby boy started flirting with me as we gulped down our cheap beer. He asked me to go outside with him to talk because the music was too loud. Naïve and buzzed on beer, I followed him outside. He led me behind a bush where no one could hear or see me. He balled his hands into fists and punched them into my shoulders, thrusting me backwards. I landed on my back so hard that the leaves on the ground ended up in my mouth and entangled in my hair. He immediately jumped on top of me, pinning me to the ground. I could not move any portion of my body. I only had my voice, knowing no one could hear or see me. I screamed, "No, get *off* me!" but this did not stop him. I knew I was going to be raped right there behind that bush.

My mind was racing with how to get out of this awful situation I had gotten myself into. I started telling him that I was going to vomit on him, pee on him, and defecate on him—anything to make myself disgusting to him. I'll never know if it was my vile words or whether someone walked near the bush, but he got off of me.

I raced back into the party and grabbed my roommate, who looked at me in shock.

"What the hell happened to you? You have leaves in your hair and dirt all over your backside!"

With tears brimming in my eyes, I told her we had to leave immediately. As we walked back to our dorm room, I sobbed, trying to recount what had just happened to me. I was baffled, confused, and scared to death. My mind could not wrap itself around why someone would do this to another human being. Because I could not understand it, my mind started justifying it. I started telling myself I drank too much. I was buzzed and couldn't make good decisions. Maybe what I wore that night was inappropriate. Shame, guilt, and secrecy flooded my racing thoughts, convincing me that this was my fault. I told no one, especially my parents, what had happened, as I knew I would be pulled out of school and sent back home to face even more turmoil. I blamed myself.

A secret and pervasive fear overtook my mind, body, and spirit that night, and it lingered for years. I spent the next four years of college escaping that fear and shame by joining a sorority, where once again I felt accepted and needed. I joined every club that would keep my mind busy and help distract from the pain and the shame. I even graduated college cum laude, again proving my self-worth.

Keeping Up with the Joneses

The endless rat race of distraction coupled with the feeling of achievement kept me at a rapid pace of doing instead of feeling, even after graduation. After college, I moved to Charlotte, North Carolina. My first job was in communications, selling pagers and cell phones. I was winning awards at work, which, in my mind, proved I was amounting to something. I gained confidence in external approvals from friends, work, and the world. But the external show was exhausting, and I found alcohol was a way to escape it all on the weekends with friends at nightclubs and parties.

Even though a fear of being raped still loomed large after my assault, alcohol continued to put me into dangerous situations. I had just started dating a semipro soccer player named Dave. He was handsome, charming, and endearing. We had only been seeing each other for a short time when he came back to my house after a night of heavy drinking. One thing led to another, and I found myself in the same position as behind that bush in college. One where I had not consented to what was happening, one where I had no control over my body, one where I felt helpless. I was date raped that evening. Once again, I was left to pick up the pieces of a shattered little girl who felt like damaged goods. I did not get out of bed for days. I missed work, I missed get-togethers with friends. The only place that felt safe was the dark hole under my comforter, where its warmth wrapped around me as my tears fell nonstop. This feeling of not being able to control the situation yet again and the helplessness I experienced left a lasting need to control almost everything else in my life thereafter.

Even though internally I felt like damaged goods, I had learned by now that my external appearance could convince the outside world otherwise. The performance must go on, despite the fact that my internal world was a disaster. As my college loans began to accumulate, I took on modeling gigs that paid good money for my appearance and the objectification of my body. It was then that I became a poster child for the alcohol industry in the most literal sense of the term.

First, I was the Budweiser Girl, strutting around bars in white high heels and a figure-hugging, short white Budweiser dress, an objectified message of what you can get if you drink Budweiser. Later, I became the Guinness Girl, where the attire was a bit more conservative, wearing a tight Guinness black T-shirt and khaki shorts. My people-pleasing and conversational skills served me well as I handed out Guinness Koozies®, endorsing their "black and tans"—half pale beer layered on top of their dark beer.

The one that still makes my stomach clench into nauseating knots is when I was the Jägermeister Girl. Adorned in another skin-tight, skimpy dress, I pranced around bars, passing out trays of little glass vials filled to the brim with Jägermeister (imagine a test tube with no lid on it). At the end of each night after my shift was over, I won shot contests, proving that I could throw back the most vials of the so-called "stag's blood."

Fortunately, a few years later, I was able to land a higher paying sales job, eliminating the side hustle of these modeling gigs. It is no surprise that I ended up taking a sales job in the aesthetics industry, where the way I looked was as important as how much I could sell. During my career in aesthetics, I fell deep into the vortex of placing my entire worth in my appearance, all while selling women on how my products could mold them into the cultural definition of beauty.

Over the next decade, the fast-paced, ever-evolving aesthetic industry started to take a toll on me. I was measured on my sales and felt I was only as good as my last quarter's numbers. My sales rankings became part of my identity, with each climb up the rankings and each award adding steam to my little engine that didn't stop hustling. This Wall Street-level pressure was met with the old saying "Work hard, play hard," in which "play" always entailed lots and lots of alcohol. It included plenty of dinners with clients at steak house restaurants, where the wine flowed freely and abundantly. And no matter what company I worked for throughout my sales career, the sales meetings were a place where we were encouraged to drink after our all-day meetings, and it was frowned upon if you didn't join the crew afterward at the bar.

Despite this pressure, I only drank on the weekends, but it was the release I needed from pushing myself all week to keep up with the Joneses. I spent my career controlling my appearance, chasing sales, winning awards, and feeling like who I was equalled what I accomplished. After years of external validation from men, work, friends, and society, I had lost who I was, what I needed, and what God intended me to be. The shame, fear, and secrecy of my past perpetuated my "not enough-ism" and the need to control all facets of my life.

Mommy Juice

By 2009, I was married with two kids and motherhood transformed my drinking into the world of "Momtinis" and enjoying good wine with friends to decompress. Through any challenges in adulthood, I turned to my old friend, alcohol, who had been by my side all these years, to escape the discomfort. After years of hearing the message "Don't feel, be happy," it had sunk in. Drink, you've *earned* it.

Drink to celebrate. Drink to relax, Momma. Drink to cope. Drink to buffer yourself from any uncomfortable feelings. Just drink, drink, *drink*.

As busy working moms who are needed at work, needed by our kids, always needed as a volunteer at school, needed as a wife, needed as a friend—I was always striving to meet everyone else's needs before my own. I could not even tell you what my own needs were. The façade, the show had to go on because stopping meant looking at what I did not want to see.

When I was growing up, my father traveled most days of the week, leaving my mom pretty much a single mother to three kids. It wasn't easy. In fact, my mom often used to tell us, "I have one drop of blood left . . . who wants it?"

After having kids of my own, I gave her a lot of credit.

Much like my mom, I would end up feeling empty at the end of my days, giving my last drop of blood to wine, and I was not a single parent. Alcohol became my permission slip to rest, check out, and find solace from all the chatter in my brain when it was telling me to do more.

Feeling like something wasn't right, I had started seeing a therapist. I learned that I had become "dutiful yet dead." I felt an enormous amount of responsibility and obligation to those in my life, but it was leaving me feeling depleted and "dead" most days. I had to "come alive" somewhere else in my life, and for me it was with alcohol—wine in particular. Mix in society's ideal of how to be the perfect mom and a successful career professional, and it all feels like there isn't enough blood in the day! I would release all the responsibilities—the need to control, the perfectionism, and the rescuing—into a rewarding glass of wine.

In Holly Whitaker's book *Quit Like a Woman*, she sums it up precisely:

> We are not only expected to be mothers, we are expected to *mother*. And not just children, *everyone*. Which is another way of saying: You are skilled at putting everyone else's needs first because our society subtly and unsubtly tells you to. As a result, you are probably not only unskilled at putting yourself first, you are probably sick from putting yourself last.[1]

As women, we have been programmed to take care of everyone else's needs first. If there is any time left, then it's for us, but there rarely is enough time. We've convinced ourselves that going to the grocery store is a break, when really it is just one more thing on our to-do list that is fulfilling everyone else's needs but our own. All day, we manage all the details that pop up for our family, combatting them like Kung Fu fighters, putting out fires, slaying after school activities and doctor appointments amidst the emails, texts, and phone calls that keep barreling at us nonstop. Then, when the day is over and our fight is won, we turn to alcohol to escape it all.

To the outside world, it looks like we have it all together; but on the inside, we are tired and exhausted by it all. Perfectionism fuels our need to control. Only when we are in control can we appear to look perfect. Alcohol, a great numbing agent, put up a strong barrier to the feelings of imperfection.

Too often, we think we need to be perfect in all aspects of our lives, when all we really need is to be real with one another. Trying to be perfect or looking like you have it all together is just perpetuating women's entrapment with alcohol. None of us are perfect. Many of us hide behind alcohol to escape this perfectionism.

When we are born, we are pure and innocent, safe in the knowledge that we are enough. Yet, slowly, as we grow up, society tells us and teaches us that we can be more, that we are *not enough*!

We constantly compare ourselves to others: at work, with rankings, promotions, and awards; in our workouts on leaderboards; and looking at our friends' seemingly perfect lives on social media. All this comparison feeds our inner critic who tells us we can do better, be more, and improve . . . just keep proving your *worth*! We yearn to belong, to be accepted, so we chip away at who we are to better fit in with everyone else. This crumbling of who we are or who we were born to be slowly diminishes over time as we build our own façade. We go with the flow of drinking, sometimes drugs, or even smoking to fit in in our adolescent years. As adults, we use alcohol, shopping, diets, and whatever we can to shape ourselves into who we think we should be, erasing and quieting that small little girl within. This seems to work in our twenties, thirties, and even longer—until it just *doesn't* anymore. Eventually you realize the mask you've fabricated isn't really working or serving you whatsoever.

What I didn't realize at the time was that I was setting myself up for a much bigger challenge with alcohol when life came crumbling down upon me.

The Lie: "I Deserve a Glass"

The Truth: The truth is we deserve to rest. From an early age, we fall prey to messages of perfectionism, not enough-ism, and over functioning to prove our worth and keep ourselves looking like we can do it all—especially in motherhood. We are pressured to drink alcohol in our adolescent years, making us more susceptible to sexual assault situations. As we move into our adult years, we fall into the trap and lie that a well-deserved drink is self-care. In reality, though, alcohol is the opposite of self-care; it makes us more anxious and depressed and separates us from ourselves. It numbs the ability to discern our own thoughts.

Did You Know?

"At least 50 percent of student sexual assaults involve alcohol. Approximately 90 percent of rapes perpetrated by an acquaintance of the victim involve alcohol. About 43 percent of sexual assault events involve alcohol use by the victim; 69 percent involve alcohol use by the perpetrator. In one-third of sexual assaults, the aggressor is intoxicated."[2]

—American Addiction Centers

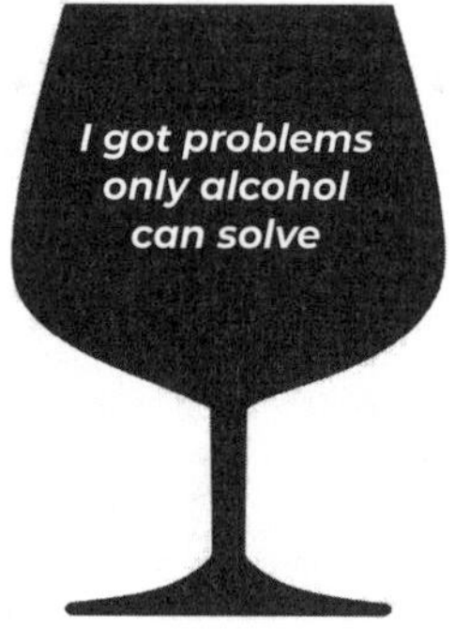

CHAPTER TWO

"YOU DON'T HAVE A DRINKING PROBLEM"

For many of us, our relationship with alcohol in early adulthood is much like a sailboat, coasting along the smooth waters at sea. We glide through parties, dinners, and celebrations with alcohol as the wind in our sails, cruising through life without giving it much thought. Then, one day out at sea, our sailboat is caught off guard by the unforeseen approach of a murky, thick, dense fog where we lose our compass and direction amongst the vast, landless sea. The fog is so thick and visibility is diminished to the point where you can no longer even see yourself. You become so disoriented, you are unable to navigate the waters ahead of you.

A few years ago, my own unforeseen, dense fog came in the form of three life-changing events that shifted my alcohol usage without my even realizing it. First, my husband, Paul, lost his job. His company was in financial distress and had been downsizing for a while. Paul was fifty years old, so we were now concerned whether he would be able to find another job within his industry. Overnight, I became the primary and sole breadwinner for our family. During this same time, we also unexpectedly lost a dear friend.

As if both of these events weren't devasting enough, another two weeks later, a close friend called to tell me she had been molested when she was younger, and she was finally ready to get justice. I became her safe person. I navigated the dark, horrifying, excruciating details of her sexual molestation encounters with her while trying to figure out how to heal both of our sexual assault pasts. I became deeply intertwined with her past as I not only wanted justice for her but also needed to heal my own past sexual injustices. I cried most evenings after work, submerged in anxiety over my husband's job loss, the raw grief and void over the loss of our beloved friend, and the all-encompassing pain and rage I felt for my friend's injustice and my own. Not knowing what to do with me, after the kids were in bed, my husband would bring a glass of wine into our room each night as tears rolled down my cheeks.

These back-to-back events catapulted me into a deep, dark place of depression, anxiety, and fear. Just like a sailboat being caught off guard in the rolling fog, these events overtook my ability to navigate a healthy relationship with alcohol. It was my nightly escape from the reality of what was really happening in my life. When I could not fix these issues, change them, or control them like I could with everything else in my past, my drinking shifted from a weekend indulgence to an almost daily occurrence. I escaped the madness in a glass of merlot. What I couldn't see was that I was numbing the good along with the bad. My days were so fogged by alcohol that I was blinded to the feelings that sat right underneath, begging to be reckoned with. Instead of feeling these feelings, I was trapped by the conditioned belief that I just needed to relax with some wine in the evenings.

Alcohol washed over all these dark feelings, numbing them away into the night. It quieted the voices that raged in my head whenever I slowed down and tried to sleep. My alcohol use was no longer recreational, it was medicinal.

What Keeps Us from Knowing

Several months later, I had begun to see a new therapist about these back-to-back events—my husband's job loss, losing our best friend unexpectedly, and becoming the safe person for a good friend—all of which were impacting and overwhelming my life. Talking with her helped, but I knew deep down something was still padding these deep, dark places, not allowing the pain to be truly felt. That small voice within was telling me something was still wrong, so I finally worked up the courage to confide in my therapist about my drinking. I sat down on her couch, rubbing my sweaty palms on my pants, searching for how to tell her my secret—or rather, my truth. I was petrified to tell her, but even more, I wanted reassurance that I wasn't crazy.

Not wasting a minute in our session, I blurted out, "I think I might have a drinking problem." There . . . it was out there. I was finally calling out my dark fear into the light. I told her about all the back and forth in my mind and how crazy I felt.

She looked at me decisively and replied, "No, no, I don't think you do. I think you are thinking about it too much."

Really? I thought. My inner knowing and that courageous voice that had been poking at me incessantly about my drinking shied back into her small, quiet place of silent submission. I felt relieved, as I trusted my therapist; she was the expert, so I doubted my own intuition once again. This time, I closed the door on my inner knowing, ignoring her pleas about my drinking behavior. Reassured that I didn't have a problem, this ill advice kept my nightly wine habit in motion for two more years.

I looked around at my friends who were all drinking what seemed to me the same amount that I was drinking, which further convinced me that I was a "normal" drinker. I wasn't blacking out all the time. I wasn't drinking during the day. I never drank to cure my hangovers. No one was in harm's way, everyone was safe. There were no external consequences related to my drinking.

But I still felt trapped in the wine cycle of hell. Like a spin cycle in the washing machine, around and around I went, often waking up in the morning groggy and disappointed for having a few once again the night before. I would spend the day working off my slight hangover with bad food choices in the morning, healthy food choices the rest of the day, coupled with a punishing, strenuous workout after work to clear out the toxins to make myself believe I was in control. Yet even after all that "undoing," I found myself again saying, "I'll only have one glass to unwind and relax."

This cycle went on for years. We know what we are doing isn't serving us, yet we go back for more. Unknowingly, each drink erases our inner knowing, dimming her, putting her in the corner, resulting in disconnection from whom we truly are, foregoing ourselves to remain in the alcohol trap with the masses.

Over the next year or so, my husband eventually found a job and my friend, though she never got justice, got her life back together.

The only person not getting better was me.

My identity was starting to collapse under the weight of my duplicity. I was winning awards at work, fulfilling my obligations as a mother and a wife, but my evenings were dedicated to what had become an almost nightly wine habit. I believed alcohol was self-care and a reward when it actually was making me sick and tired. I felt like there was an a.m. me and a p.m. me. During the day when alcohol was not present, I felt in total control; then, just as the sun set, something would shift in my brain asking, pleading, begging for a space where there was no control. A complete release. That sense of release brought darkness in the shape of blurred nights, arguments with my husband, and hours away from my kids that were wasted in the bottle.

There would be days I wouldn't drink, so I thought I was okay. Occasionally, I would stop drinking for a few days, sometimes two weeks, but it was always sheer willpower that got me through. White knuckling it always gave way to fatigue and ultimately caving once again. After not drinking for a while and convincing myself I did not have a problem, I would just fall further into the bottle when I drank again. My drinking always came back with a vengeance after taking a break. I felt captive in a purgatory of gray.

I am exhausted. I need to escape and check out.
I deserve a drink . . . just one drink to unwind.
I'll just have one more . . .
My Vicious Drinking and Shame Cycle
I wake up riddled with anxiety at 3 a.m., fall back to sleep, then wake up to star my day feeling groggy, tired, and in a fog.
Shouldn't have had so much to drink. Why do I do this?
I need to make this right with a workout and healthy food.
I feel better now. See, I am fine. I am in control.
I did everything on my to-do list and took care of everyone's needs.

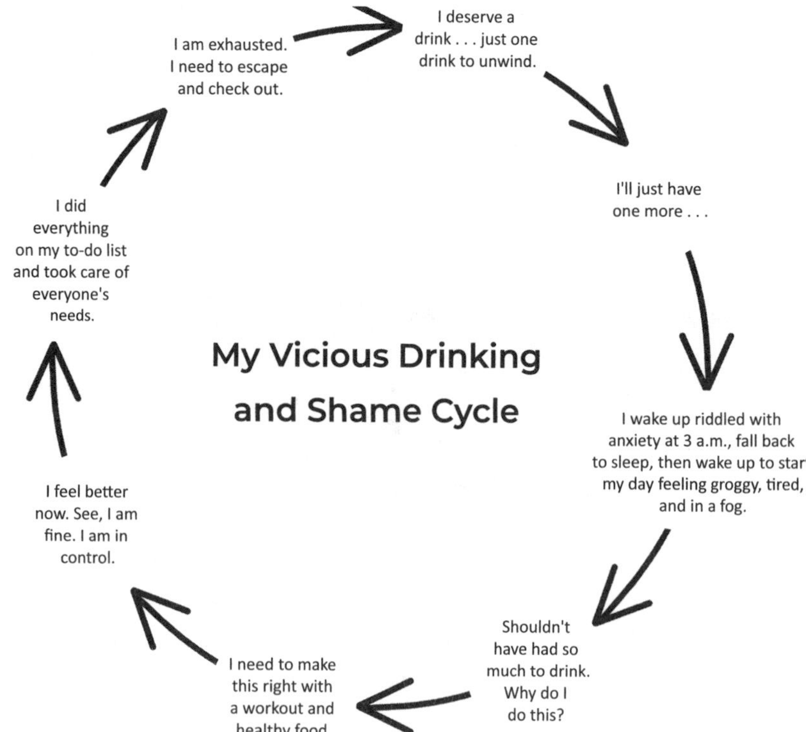

Shame and Shoulds

The worst part of my drinking was the shame that came along with it. I was trapped in a vicious shame cycle of *I should have done this, but I did that.* Shame is another lie we buy into. Some of us were even told when we were younger, "Shame on you." Shame makes us feel bad about our actions and that we are not good enough. Shame is something we quietly struggle with in our heads, beating ourselves up, and around and around we go. We punish ourselves or try to fix our wrongdoings, and that puts our perfectionism into overdrive, leading us to believe that we are in control once again.

One night, my husband and I went out to a bar in our beach town. It was the anniversary of the passing of our beloved friend. There was so much heartache and grief we couldn't even articulate, so we drowned it all out in several drinks. After one too many, we came home to our condominium where our ten- and fourteen-year-old kids were waiting for us. I clumsily stumbled in my wedged heels when I walked through the front door. The kids thought it was funny and started videotaping me on their cell phones. I kept telling them that if they did not stop, I would take their cell phones away—then I started to count to ten. The problem was I kept repeating myself over and over counting to ten, threatening them, to the point where it was ridiculous and nonsensical.

I woke up the next morning with the most horrific hangover. The kids came into my bedroom and said, "Mom, you were *so* drunk last night. You kept repeating yourself. You kept threatening to take our cell phones. Look, look at this video."

Bleary eyed and buried in embarrassment, I watched their video of me stumbling into a wall then onto my bed, repeating exactly what they said I had said. Shame engulfed my throbbing head. Immediately, I started to beat myself up. *Why did I drink so much last night*? More shameful thoughts started to flood in: *You are not a good parent. You were a mess and your kids saw it. What are you modeling to them*? *You should have drunk less; you know better.*

We all know that children just want to feel safe. I knew I had crossed the line with my behavior. I knew something *had* to change.

My coping mechanisms that always tricked me into believing I was in control of my drinking were no longer convincing me that I was fine. I had Googled *Do I have a drinking problem*? so many times that my computer was convinced I did. I knew deep down I wasn't thinking about it too much; I knew I needed help.

Twenty-One Days to Reveal the Truth

Right around this time, I stumbled upon an ad on Facebook for a 21-Day Reset Challenge to evaluate your relationship with alcohol. At first, I ignored the ad for a few months, reminding myself of what my therapist had said—that I was thinking about it too much. But that small inner voice was relentless. The little girl I had banished poked her head out again, begging me to listen to her. I finally clicked on the Sober Sis ad, finding a community of like-minded women who also felt they needed to explore their relationship with alcohol and its impact on their lives. It was a judgment-free, online group of women from all over the world questioning their relationship with alcohol . . . just like me.

Jenn Kautsch, founder of Sober Sis, coined a great phrase: the "detox just to retox" loop.[1] And it spoke right to the core of my struggle. Jenn describes "the detox" as doing everything healthy, mindful, and responsible by day only to turn around and seemingly undo it by mindless sipping, living on autopilot, and making choices from a divided mind . . . one that is in contrast to your true goals. The loop begins again the next morning with good intentions only to be undone—yet again—by evening.[2]

They say it takes 21 days to change a habit or start a new one. Sober Sis pledged that after the 21-Day Reset, I would never look at alcohol in quite the same way again.

That was Halloween 2019.

Perfect, I thought, *I will just do this online 21-Day Reset or "No-Alcohol November" challenge to get my drinking back on track.* I was still convinced and stuck in thinking I could control this highly celebrated, highly addictive drug. I figured I had let my guard down, and since everyone around me could apparently control it, I just needed a few tools to reign it back in with everyone else.

I was excited to get the tools to find a way back to "drinking responsibly" (whatever that means). We were put into a group of thirty-two women on a video app called Marco Polo (a back-and-forth online video platform) where we could discuss our daily lessons on being alcohol-free. I was surprised to see women ranging from twenty-one to eighty years old taking part. *Alcohol doesn't care about age*, I thought, *but it's never too early or too late to begin your exploration.*

I heard someone once say, "Fear cannot survive in a safe place where it is called out." This is what my Sober Sis group became to me: A safe place to question my fears. A place to look at my vulnerabilities in the light with other women whom I had never met but who were divinely similar to me in so many ways. Together, we listened to each other's stories of what brought us to this exploration. And when we first started making our online videos on Marco Polo, the cultural expectation of perfectionism was glaring at us on our phones.

The first thing many of the women would say when they got on Marco Polo was "I look terrible today" or "I don't have any makeup on." The self-deprecation would continue with "Excuse my tired look" or "I look horrible." Only then they would begin sharing their vulnerable stories of what brought them to Sober Sis.

I got on after several of these introductions and said, "Ladies, we need to stop getting on here and saying 'I look terrible' as our opening comment. No one cares! We only care about your authenticity and vulnerability that allows us to see the true you and connects us to one another."

Marco Polo was an ironically powerful social media tool, literally forcing us to look at ourselves on our phone, facing the truest version of ourselves: messy yet beautiful—perfect, though we hardly felt like it. It was a tool that allowed each of us to practice voicing our truth when our voices were lost in a bottle.

We let the secrets that fueled our shame and guilt over the years dissipate by being real and authentic about our relationship with alcohol with one another. We realized how we all were using it as a reward at the end of the day, to fill a void, escape a pain or trauma, or "enhance" our fun social gatherings or celebrations. We left our judgments of perfectionism—who we should have been and what we were supposed to be—offline and showed up for each other virtually, seeing the beauty in the mess.

The messes we shared online connected us deeply and quickly. What would normally have taken years to develop into true friendships was happening instantaneously for us over Marco Polo. We had support in our pockets, on our cell phones, allowing us at a moment's notice to jump on for help and understanding. We were strangers who shared our darkest points in life and bravely came together to support one another in ways we hadn't even experienced with our own lifelong friends. Within a few days, our deep connection and nonjudgmental support made us feel like we had known each other all our lives.

Throughout this book, I'd like to introduce you to some of the women from my Sober Sis group—women who, just like you and me, realized that something wasn't right in their relationship with alcohol. Women who linked arms in busting and debunking the deceptions of alcohol.

Read these words from Lisa, Betsy, Elizabeth, Stacy, and Anna and see if you can identify with their sense of unease:

> ***Lisa***: I drank from the age of fifteen, but it was always for fun, at parties and events. I did notice that I always drank more than my friends, but that's just "who I was." I had fun. But when I turned fifty, a family crisis dealing with my daughter took me to the phase that I struggled with for over a decade. I needed something to take away the pain. I simply could not deal with this. I, who was referred to by my friends and work associates as "Wonder Woman," could not take this pain for one more second. That was the first time I deliberately went home to purposely get drunk to get numb. What a relief.
>
> Over the next ten years, I saw my daughter sink lower and lower in her own life, but I dealt with it every evening, preferably by myself. "How can you handle it?" people would ask when they saw me completely put together at school, volunteering, writing a book, building a house, or celebrating wedding anniversaries. "How do you do it?" And my pat answer was that I had a lot of people praying for me every day. The truth was that I had a chilled bottle of wine waiting for me every evening.

Betsy: I think I was a gray area drinker the moment I started drinking because I never drank in high school but started drinking in college. My drinking was a social, binge-type drinking on the weekends. I always drank with other people; it was a social thing for me. Then, after college, I continued to be a social drinker except during my pregnancies. It was easy to stop when I was pregnant or on a diet or a cleanse. But when I did drink, I always overdrank. It was always detoxing until the next social event . . . it wasn't everyday drinking.

I never thought my drinking was abnormal because everyone was cutting loose like me. They may have been cutting loose from time to time, but I was cutting loose *every* time. I was a straight A student, had a very successful career, raised my kids—I don't think anyone would have thought I had a problem with alcohol. Later, when struggling through some adjustments of midlife, I found myself drinking alone. That scared me more than not having an "off switch." That's when I started to examine my relationship with alcohol. I joined our group to get back to just social drinking.

Elizabeth: I knew I had a problem when I went to the zoo with my kids where they were selling beer and mixed slushy alcoholic drinks . . . and I was excited. I was thinking, *This is great*! *They have alcohol at the zoo*! I wanted to have a drink in the afternoon . . . at the *zoo*! It hit me like, *What is wrong with me*? *Why am I drinking beer at the zoo*? It got me thinking: I was thinking about it too much.

Stacy: Strangely enough, the switch flipped on me, and I had to adjust to a new normal. In five years, my three children left home. Just like that, I was empty nested. The crazy schedule of attending performances, meetings, celebrations, waiting up, and having a house filled with teenagers was over. It was dead quiet. And while worry about my "adult-ish" children actually adulting often made my stomach flip, I felt like I had been fired from a job I had done wholeheartedly for twenty-five years. I was now expected to stay quiet and let them fly, fall, and figure out the lessons of life. The super-fast hamster wheel had just stopped. I fell off with a jolt, and now my life had a very empty calendar. Literally. No everyday connections and lunches with the other moms to stay in the loop, no tech rehearsals to attend for costume checks, no games on tap for the weekends, no late-night and early-morning debriefs of the latest romantic and friend dramas. No trying to balance my part-time design jobs . . . none of that. Just quiet. And a lot of time on my hands to grapple with my identity.

The "wine witch" can so easily come flying in wanting to help ease the ache, the loneliness, the empty time. So *much* empty time. A poor counselor to say "Wow, all you thought you needed was time to work on you, and now you are lost in the journey."

I often feel I don't have the heart to look for that girl who has been buried under all of those busy days that led to weeks that led to years.

> ***Anna***: I too felt alcohol was in control of me. I found myself on Halloween finding any excuse to go back home to drink my wine—like I needed to let the dogs out or go to the bathroom—just so I could get back to the refrigerator and grab some more wine.

All of these women's stories are different but the same, underscoring the struggle so many have with their relationship with alcohol. We were all concerned how much we were becoming a slave to the drink. We were concerned about how much we were thinking about alcohol and how we were using it as self-care.

Amanda Doyle, sister of podcast host Glennon Doyle and cohost of *We Can Do Hard Things*, once said, "I got a package in the mail the other day that was a set of wine glasses that said 'SELF-CARE' on them . . . that isn't self-care. The actual wine is not the self-care. The time with your friends is self-care. If the only self-care you are giving yourself is wine, what you are accepting as self-care is a shitty consolation prize to what actually is self-care."[3]

It's confusing, though, when your self-care and slave-to-the-bottle behavior are being reinforced as normal and the way to unwind and rest by those around you. We see our friends with their insulated drink coolers concealing a coveted alcoholic drink at football games, amusement parks, playdates, and so on. Memes on social media encouraging us to drink to deal with life's ups and downs only further this thought process. Television shows and movies glamourizing and romanticizing alcohol reinforce it by putting alcohol on a pedestal. In our reset program, all of us realized and learned we had fallen into the trap of gray area drinking, something I had never heard of before.

What Is Gray Area Drinking?

In my mind, either you had to hit rock bottom with your drinking, or you were a "normal" drinker. In my Sober Sis program, I learned many of the women identified with a term called gray area drinking. I don't like labels, but so many of us are trapped here that if we don't learn to call it what it is, we will only continue to fall prey to it. By listening to the women in my Sober Sis group's various drinking stories, I had discovered that gray area drinking comes in many shades of gray. Your drinking may fall into a lighter or darker hue of gray, but it is still a problem. As Aidan Donnelley Rowley, cohost of *Editing Our Drinking and Our Lives* podcast, says, "It may have been a lowercase 'p' problem, but it was still a problem."[4]

I want to reiterate: I am not here to diagnose anyone. My hope is that by sharing some statistics from the medical and sober community in conjunction with my story, it will allow you to see whether you fit into this category and help you explore your relationship with alcohol.

Often, as a society, we want to put people in boxes, to label them to make ourselves feel better. We want a clear checklist to make sure we don't have a problem. But gray area drinking is not clear; it's this murky, thick, vast, no-end-in-sight, perplexing middle space. Even the dictionary depicts how difficult a "gray area" is to discern: The *Merriam-Webster Dictionary* defines a gray area as "an area or situation in which it is difficult to judge what is right and what is wrong."[5]

Jolene Park, a TED speaker and the leading authority on gray area drinking, defines gray area drinking as follows:

> Gray area drinking is the space between end-stage drinking and every now and again drinking.
>
> It's a large spectrum.
>
> It's self-identified.
>
> It doesn't take a huge amount of alcohol to become a gray area drinker because . . . there is no safe or recommended healthy intake level of alcohol.
>
> It often involves years of inner questioning and inner struggle more than other consequences.
>
> It's very common. Especially among women.
>
> It's the ability to stop drinking without needing a medical detox, but it's hard to stay stopped.
>
> It's a problem for many people.
>
> It's one of the biggest public health epidemics of our time. Thankfully, more and more people are stepping off the gray area drinking merry-go-round and talking about it publicly which inspires others to do the same.
>
> It's about quitting drinking because you choose to, not because you have to.[6]

Alcoholism exists on a continuum called the spectrum of alcohol use disorder (AUD), which ranges from mild to moderate to severe. On one end of the spectrum, there are the individuals who abstain from drinking altogether. Then there are those in the "mild" category who drink on occasion, who have a few from time to time.

Gray area drinkers end up somewhere in the "moderate-to-severe" part of the spectrum. These drinkers rarely can just have one. They may take breaks for days or weeks, but at some point, they always go back to their old ways. On the far end of the spectrum are those diagnosed with alcoholism, which falls into the "severe" area, drinkers who are physically and psychologically dependent on alcohol.

To show just how difficult it is to concretely quantify the gray area drinking space on the AUD spectrum, here are just a couple definitions of gray area drinking: The National Institute on Alcohol Abuse and Alcoholism (NIAAA) defines low-risk drinking as fourteen or fewer drinks per week and four or fewer drinks on any day for men and seven or fewer drinks per week and three or fewer drinks on any day for women.[7]

Yet an article in the *Journal of Studies on Alcohol and Drugs* defines gray area consumption as men who drank fourteen or fewer drinks per week and four or fewer drinks on any given day but who drank more than two drinks on at least one day and women who drank seven or fewer drinks per week and three or fewer drinks on any day but who drank more than one drink on at least one day.[8]

Confusing, isn't it? To the outside world, no one can tell as this agonizing tug of war rages within your head. No wonder there is so much confusion surrounding gray area drinking when there aren't any negative external consequences that clearly signal you need help. Most of us look like we have our shit together. Highly functioning go-getters . . . at work, at home, and in our personal lives. As Jolene Park states in her popular 2017 TED talk on gray area drinking, many of her gray area drinking clients are CEOs, lawyers, and highly successful entrepreneurs who are functioning well in society but struggling quietly.[9]

Gray area drinking is an isolated place that leaves you wondering: *What is wrong with me? Why can't I get this under control like everyone else?*

It is even more confusing because, as a society, we tend to measure by the number of drinks, not even considering the number of ounces. And you might be surprised to learn how little truly moderate drinking actually is. The US Dietary Guidelines for Americans, for example, recommends that those who drink do so in moderation. They define moderation as one drink per day for women and two drinks per day for men.[10] Also, consider that a standard glass of wine is five ounces, but many people pour much, *much* more.

I can tell you most of my glasses were not five ounces. I would trick myself into believing I did not have that much by only counting the glasses, *never* the ounces. Most restaurant pours are rarely ever five ounces. This counting of glasses versus ounces only reinforces our belief that we don't have a problem.

Do I Have a Problem?

It has been said that if you are not questioning your relationship with alcohol (like I was), you probably don't have a problem with it. While there's no concrete checklist to tell you whether you fall into gray area drinking, read these signs of gray area drinking below from some various sources to see if they resonate with you:

Ria Health Website (Riahealth.com)

- You feel concerned about your drinking, but you can never seem to quit permanently.
- You haven't experienced any life-shattering problems because of alcohol. But in the back of your mind, you still worry about it.
- You drink to deal with emotions—i.e., you'll have a mixed drink after work every night to cope with stress.
- Alcohol is an integrated habit in your life. It almost seems unfathomable to go out with friends or relax after dinner without having a couple of drinks.[11]

Jolene Park's Website (Grayareadrinkers.com)

- You don't experience outward consequences from drinking but struggle internally.
- You have silent conversations with yourself about your own drinking.
- You intend to have one glass of wine but find it all too easy to finish the whole bottle.
- You stop drinking, for weeks or even months, then restart again, because "Why be so restrictive?"
- You realize the way you're drinking isn't helping you have the life you want.[12]

Jenn Kautsch's Sober Sis Website (Sobersis.com/ss-home)

- Over time, I've found myself drinking more but enjoying it less. Often, I'm just drinking mindlessly out of habit.
- Sometimes I feel so anxious, and I think alcohol might be making it worse.
- I equate a drink(s) at wine o'clock to transition to being "off duty." It feels like a reward and something I think about throughout the day.
- I am drinking to "take the edge off," but I fear that I'm losing my edge because my brain is so foggy.
- I justify my drinking by comparing myself to others . . . always normalizing it or measuring myself to someone worse. I feel stuck.[13]

If you suspect from these indicators that you might fall somewhere in the gray area drinking category—or even if you think, like I did, you don't have a problem at all—the National Institute on Alcohol Abuse and Alcoholism (NIAAA) has created a definitive list of questions that providers might use to see if you exhibit symptoms of alcohol use disorder (AUD). These questions can be a helpful self-check for those of us wondering if we might be falling prey to the lies of alcohol.

Ask yourself: In the past year, have you

- Had times when you ended up drinking more, or longer, than you intended?
- More than once wanted to cut down or stop drinking, or tried to, but couldn't?
- Spent a lot of time drinking? Or being sick or getting over other aftereffects?
- Wanted a drink so badly you couldn't think of anything else?
- Found that drinking—or being sick from drinking—often interfered with taking care of your home or family? Or caused job troubles? Or school problems?
- Continued to drink even though it was causing trouble with your family or friends?
- Given up or cut back on activities that were important or interesting to you, or gave you pleasure, in order to drink?
- More than once gotten into situations while or after drinking that increased your chances of getting hurt (such as driving, swimming, using machinery, walking in a dangerous area, or having unprotected sex)?
- Continued to drink even though it was making you feel depressed or anxious or adding to another health problem? Or after having had a memory blackout?
- Had to drink much more than you once did to get the effect you want? Or found that your usual number of drinks had much less effect than before?

- Found that when the effects of alcohol were wearing off, you had withdrawal symptoms, such as trouble sleeping, shakiness, restlessness, nausea, sweating, a racing heart, or a seizure? Or sensed things that were not there?[14]

When I started on my sober-curious journey, I could answer yes to several of these questions, landing me on the "moderate" area on the AUD spectrum. As part of our healthcare evaluations with our primary care physicians, we are only asked if we drink and how many drinks per week, but we are rarely asked for more descriptive details about our drinking lives, adding to the confusion and stigma of black-and-white drinking. Because I never hit a rock bottom, it was a tricky mind game in the middle. One where society told me I was a "normal" drinker and that, in fact, I was handling the stress of life the right way—with a drink. Many people told me that they did not think I had a problem with drinking, including my own therapist. Needless to say, she is no longer my therapist.

We look to our healthcare professionals, therapists, and wellness instructors for guidance on our drinking behavior and are often told by these experts, it is fine. It adds to our confusion when our minds are questioning our behavior. I recently took a spin class where the fitness instructor talked about being hungover and even said, "You may even still be drunk. It is okay, sweat out the toxins!"

And we wonder why we have divided minds!

Pro-drinking messages are subtly inserted into our conversations with experts who we look up to—allowing these messages to normalize our gray area drinking. We do not talk about eating pizza during our workout class, so why should we hear about drinking? If we don't stop to question these things, then they become part of our identity.

Sober Sis Founder Jenn Kautsch paints the perfect picture of gray area drinking: "It is like a one-way drinking highway: It's only going in one direction. Where you are on the highway is different for everyone and you might take an earlier exit ramp or later exit ramp."[15]

Expanding upon her analogy, as we drive down this one-way drinking highway, we see warning signs such as "More Blackouts Ahead" or "Caution: Drinking Alone Around the Bend," but often we ignore these warning signs, heading further down a dead-end street. Some of us see the warning signs and then take the exit ramp to take a break from drinking (like "Dry January"), only to merge back onto the highway later. This starting and stopping only adds to the confusion of gray area drinking.

Debunking "Rock Bottom"

So why do we think we have to hit a rock bottom in order to examine our relationship with alcohol? We hear and see the horror stories from friends, in books, on TV, and in movies of someone who has hit rock bottom from their "problematic" or "high-risk" drinking. We might see on TV a character who has been told they should, or perhaps even been forced to, get help as a result of their drinking. We are told to "drink responsibly" (again, whatever that means) or "to drink in moderation" by controlling our alcohol or at least appearing like we can to the outside world. One more show, one more act . . . trapping us into silence.

Kari Schwear, founder of GrayTonic and the Question the Drink® movement, says, "For far too long, society has placed problematic drinking in a black or white box. One is *either* an alcoholic or they are not. That is simply not true. About 50 percent of people who consume alcohol are in the gray area."[16]

We are also taught to fear alcoholism and the stigma associated with it. This fear is kept at bay by the normative drinking culture in which gray area drinking feels normal and is accepted by our peers. I never had anyone tell me "I think you should get help" or "Maybe you should talk to someone about your drinking." It was just the opposite. When I asked loved ones, "Do you think I drink too much?" I never got one response back in the affirmative. In fact, when I shared my idea to join an online group exploring my relationship with alcohol, it was always met from loved ones with a resounding "I never felt like you had a problem" or "Do you think you were addicted?"

This black-and-white projection on our drinking behavior kept me trapped in gray area drinking for years. I found myself baffled at why I felt this incredible tug of war raging in my head with my alcohol usage, but no one around me seemed to be questioning their alcohol usage like I was, so I blamed myself. I figured *I* had a problem. It was *my* issue. It was an isolating and lonely place of suffering, shame, and guilt.

Identifying and relating to the gray area drinking category created the space and the capacity for me to explore my relationship with alcohol with a group of sober-curious women who felt just like I did. I was beginning to see through the fog and those gray hues to a place where stories like mine resonated with my inner knowing. It became clear, the bigger question was not "Do I have a drinking problem?" but rather "What is drinking doing for me?" If our gray area drinking looks normal, I began to wonder why there were thousands of women in my group questioning their relationship with alcohol just like me. And maybe just like you.

The Costs of Gray Area Drinking

For overwhelmed mothers caught in gray area drinking, we constantly complain that there isn't enough time in our day, yet we drink down the seductive lies of alcohol for hours, only to have it slow us down the next day.

When our children are young, we rush through bedtime stories to get back to our much-deserved glass of wine. Or we are too checked out to read the entire book, so we summarize the bedtime stories, hoping our children will not notice. Sadly, these nighttime routines pass by quickly and we miss out on cherished moments with our young children—all for a drink. When they are older, we may find ourselves rushing to get home from baseball practice or a dance recital so we can celebrate with our favorite beverage. And, sadly, some of us attended these functions with wine in our Yetis and refills in the cooler.

The irony of all this is the "twenty-minute rule." Twenty minutes is the numbing-out period, or relaxation time, we get from drinking alcohol. Beyond twenty minutes, we are just trying to chase that feeling.

Annie Grace, author of *This Naked Mind*, shared this rule with her followers on social media, stating, "Alcohol only gives you a twenty-minute high . . . after that dopamine release, we sink lower than before." She goes on to say, "It only takes twenty minutes to sit with your emotions that will pass in twenty minutes or less as well."[17]

I was drinking for hours for just twenty minutes of escape! I did not realize that if I had just sat with my emotions for twenty minutes or less, they would have passed. What an absolute time suck!

Another steep cost of gray area drinking is forgetting meaningful conversations with loved ones. The cost of that loss of connection is one on which you cannot put a price. Trying to remember—

and act—like they recalled stories with loved ones was too costly for many of the women in my group. This is especially damaging to our children who need to feel heard and acknowledged. It's an awful feeling when you can't remember the details of their conversations due to alcohol-induced amnesia!

I am not one to count the days, but our group found an app that showed the shocking stats since we gave up the drink on November 1, 2019. As I write this, we had all saved well over $13,600 and more than 272,092 calories by giving up the drink! We had gained over 2,700 productivity hours—can you say *timesaver*?! And most nauseating of all, if we were still drinking on average, we would have consumed over 2,720 drinks in this time period.

Yuck!

The physical cost took a toll on me daily. I would wake up at a deficit, working all day trying to get back to normal. The mental anguish left me in a daily shame cycle coupled with a silent back-and-forth struggle, a war within my head that had no end in sight. The loss of freedom and feeling trapped was the biggest cost of all. I was sick and tired of being sick and tired.

The Lie: "You Don't Have a Drinking Problem"

The Truth: The problem is not you, it's alcohol, a highly addictive drug. You are not alone. You are not crazy. The lie we are told by our alcohol-centric society is that a drink will solve our problems, but deep down we know this is not true. Our problems are still there after we guzzle down the lies. Once we can see through the illusions of gray area drinking, we can see how alcohol is impacting our lives. Getting curious about our relationship with alcohol diminishes the fear and uncertainty surrounding it. Finding similar stories, other women, and a community where you can relate to their drinking is key in your sober-curious journey.

Did You Know?

"Alcohol changes levels of serotonin and other neurotransmitters in the brain, which can worsen anxiety. In fact, you may feel more anxious after the alcohol wears off. Alcohol-induced anxiety can last for several hours or even for an entire day after drinking."[18]

—Healthline

It's not really
drinking alone
if your kids are
at home

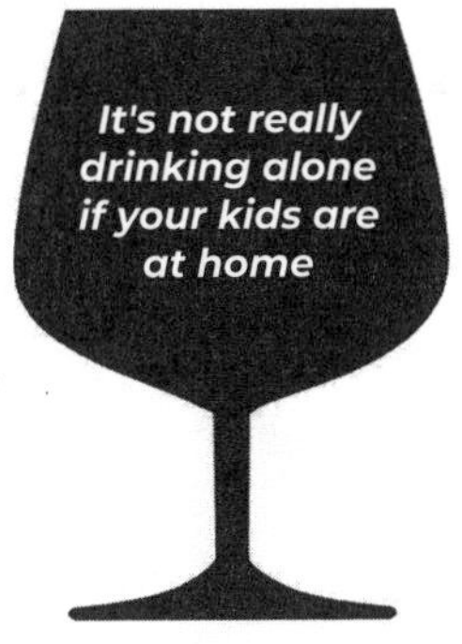

CHAPTER THREE

"I CAN CONTROL MY DRINKING"

During my 21-Day Reset without alcohol, my cravings for wine heckled me like a cackling witch. They were almost unbearable! The wine witch's flight schedule always started around dinnertime in my house, laughing as she flew past me in the kitchen, crowing, *Come on, my pretty, you can have just one glass of wine . . . hee-hee*. For parents of little ones, the "witching hours" are commonly known as the hours between dinner and bedtime. It's a time where everyone is exhausted, overstimulated, and cranky from the day. I used to drink after these hours as a way to survive them. Now they were my hardest hours to abstain from alcohol.

The onset of "me time" paired with the view of my wine bottles, a symbol of the end of my day, always triggered intense cravings.

A few days into my reset, I had just made a big Italian dinner while my husband made a roaring fire in our fireplace. The perfect time to unwind with a big glass of merlot. Every inch of my body screamed, *Just one, you can do it! Just one glass of wine in front of the warm fire—you deserve it. You don't drink* that *much! You've got this*!

I knew in my heart it wouldn't be just one glass. I knew I would feel like crap in the morning, unlike feeling better without alcohol the last few days. I reminded myself of what I had just learned in my reset, that it takes seven to ten days for alcohol to completely leave your body. Did I really want to start this all over again?

Most of the women in my Sober Sis group—not all, but the majority—found wine to be their drink of choice. As Glennon Doyle, author of *Untamed* and podcast host of *We Can Do Hard Things*, says in her fifth episode, "Wine is the opiate for women."[1]

As my "opiate" was trying to lure my brain with seductive lies to come on back, I quickly jumped online with my Sober Sisters and posted on Marco Polo: "It's the 5 p.m. witching hour and she is a real bitch tonight. I just want one glass of red wine with my nice warm fire and delicious meal, but I am coming on here to hold myself accountable. I am going to make myself a fabulous mocktail instead."

There . . . it was out there now. No going back. The thought of having to tell my group I had fallen back into the alcohol trap was not an option for me. I knew I had to reign it in, and for me that was abstaining completely during those twenty-one days. I was still caught up in the perfection show, where I wanted to prove to myself that I had my drinking under control.

But I had done more than that, more than just not drink one night. I had officially and successfully "surfed the crave" and held myself accountable. Surfing the crave meant I had observed my craving and experienced it without engaging in it. I had banished the wine witch from my house that evening with the support of my group, a mocktail, and a plan. I played it forward by visualizing what I would do and how I would feel, knowing wine would not serve me.

All the women jumped on Marco Polo, responding, holding me accountable, offering support, and asking for the same for themselves. There was an overwhelming feeling of validation and being seen in our Marco Polo group. We were no longer alone in this silent struggle. Our fears were cast out into the light together. Knowing these women had my back, I woke up the next morning feeling clear-minded, full of energy, and stronger mentally. I thought, *I can do this.*

> Dopamine is a chemical released in the brain that makes you feel good. Having the right amount of dopamine is important both for your body and your brain. Dopamine is responsible for allowing you to feel pleasure, satisfaction, and motivation. When you feel good that you have achieved something, it's because you have a surge of dopamine in the brain. It's possible, however, that you start craving more of this dopamine 'reward', which is caused by many pleasant experiences, including eating nice food, having sex, winning a game, and earning money. Alcohol and many illegal drugs cause a surge of dopamine too, which is partly why people get addicted to them.[2]
>
> —Health Direct

The first few weeks of abstaining from alcohol were also met with intense cravings for sugar. The house was still loaded full of Halloween candy, and I was literally like a kid in a candy store.

I never ate dessert in all my years of drinking. Now, over two weeks into being alcohol-free, I found myself eating a bag of gummy bears a day as my brain searched for that nightly dopamine hit.

My intense sugar cravings were also met with sleepless nights during my detox period. My body was accustomed to falling asleep to the wine lullaby. I had convinced myself that I needed the wine to quiet the monkey mind that started racing the moment my head hit the pillow. I used to tell myself that alcohol was surely better than taking Ambien. I would fall asleep easily with the down regulation wine brought over my nervous system. But it was just another illusion alcohol had told my brain. I would wake up in the middle of the night with a dry mouth, anxious thoughts, and the urgent need to pee. I cannot remember a single night of good sleep after a night of drinking.

Author William Porter explains this struggle with sleep and alcohol in his book *Alcohol Explained*:

> In a natural cycle of sleep, you will have six or seven cycles of REM sleep. However, when you drink, you will typically only have two. The reason for this is that when we drink, we go into a very deep sleep for the first five hours or so. You would be forgiven for thinking that this is a good thing, as we would usually associate a deep sleep with an invigorating and refreshing sleep, but this is not the case. The initial five hours or so of drinking sleep do not have enough REM sleep.[3]

To help with my sleeping issues, I decided to join a nightly meditation class online. I had never meditated before my alcohol-free journey but had heard its calming effects would help me sleep. Each night, I logged onto the online meditation class with my body, brain, and spirit entangled from the day's stresses and nothing to numb it any longer. Slowly, the instructor's soothing, guiding voice would unwind my clenched body and spirit. I would unravel the day's stress, letting it go in each breath. I felt grounded and calm, with a peace that washed over me before bed. I started to learn how to fall asleep again on my own.

Headaches were also a regular occurrence during my detox period. I never really got them before, other than the throbbing hangover headaches that would soon be soothed away with comfort food. I was also eating more, as my brain tried to replace eating with the calming effects I had received from alcohol with food instead.

At the beginning of my journey, abstaining from alcohol left me wondering if I had made the right choice. Could I really do this, and how long would this not-so-great feeling last?

Reading *This Naked Mind* by Annie Grace coupled with my Sober Sis daily lessons was paramount to getting me through this initial phase. Both exposed the naked truth about alcohol and all its dangers that were covered up and romanticized by our society. I learned that everything I was experiencing was normal. I honored my body going through this transition by not restricting it with a diet or quitting coffee at the same time I was trying to become alcohol-free. I met my body where it was and honored what it needed to remain alcohol-free. Thankfully, the sleepless nights, headaches, and intense sugar cravings passed shortly thereafter.

Why Quit?

As time progressed, the thought of drinking still crept up on most of us at 5 p.m., like the ocean tugging us with its undercurrent to see if we would allow it to sweep us out to sea. The pull and tug were so great, it almost felt impossible to make it to the shore of being alcohol-free. I still wasn't convinced that I wanted to be alcohol-free permanently, but I had to start digging deep to even make it through those first twenty-one days.

Just as surfers know they must swim through the wave to avoid being pummeled, some of us in our Sober Sis group chose to dive into the wave, swimming through our addiction to the other side. Other women were stuck in the foamy, turbulent water, not being able to see why they stopped in the first place. It was a daily pull and tug, push and pull that had to be met with a resounding *why* we wanted to stop.

In order to put my anchor down in this turbulent sea, I had to learn what my why was to being alcohol-free, coupled with the "what" that drove me to drink in the first place.

I began journaling every morning on why I wanted to possibly not drink. I took inventory of what I thought alcohol was doing for—and to—my life. I journaled about what I really wanted in my life, how I was feeling, and the truths about alcohol that were revealed to me since I began my exploration. Here is an entry from my journal in November 2019:

> In the beginning, stopping drinking is much like the trees and the changing seasons. As we exit fall and enter winter, another change is upon us. We are like trees: our whys on quitting drinking are like the roots of the tree, anchored deep within the earth. The storms of life will come trying to knock you over, but your deep-rooted why keeps you grounded.
>
> Your leaves start to change color as you see parts of yourself that you have not seen before as you become alcohol-free. This change is beautiful, showcasing your bright reds, yellows, and oranges, showing off who you

> truly are. As these shifts occur, you shed your old leaves off, leaving you barren. Your exposed branches feel sensitive, feeling all the feels. The chill in the air, the sting in the frost. Trees lose their leaves purposefully so when the cold winter winds blow, the branches are barren to sway in the wind. As the leaves fall to the ground, they twist and turn, spinning to the ground.
>
> Going through these transitions can feel much like leaves giving way, spinning to the ground. In time, you grow new buds and new leaves of a new you, giving shade and protection to your well-rooted trunk. You begin to learn how to nurture yourself. Now when the winds of life blow, you gently bend, allowing them to give way to the beautiful rays of sunshine and all life has to offer.

Your why must be so deeply rooted that when the choice to drink arises again, it may bend, but it does not break, as it has been planted so deeply into the earth, tethering you to your choice to not drink. Each morning hangover-free brings more life to your why, snuggled within the earth, allowing its roots to grow further and further down into the ground. The rain nourishes the root, and even though it feels dark, it strengthens the root amidst the pain. The pain shows us that when we allow our vulnerability to show up, it diminishes our fears, and we can grow deeper into the earth's soil. So when the storms of life unleash their relentless wind and rain upon you, grow taller and stronger in the choice you have made.

My why is to be the healthiest and best version of myself. My why is to be an attentive, clear-minded mother to my children and my family. My why is to be who God designed me to be, not a façade.

Early on, my dad instilled a seed of faith in me. He always had sticky notes posted all over his house, reaffirming God's love for us and the need to love *ourselves.* Over time, these seeds grew my intention for my life. For me, my truth is that we are all connected, we are all one. God, the Universe, the Divine or whatever higher power you ascribe to—for me, these are all one. I am one with the Universe, with God's love for me and all of us. I am firmly planted in His greater purpose and His desire for me to be an expression of His love. In order to be His expression, I need to be clear-minded, present, and not blurred or fogged out. I know His desire is for me to be the best version of myself, and I cannot do that with alcohol obscuring what He wants me to learn and be.

Your why must be your anchor; otherwise, the storms of life will push you back into the waves of turbulent water, leaving you confused and lost. My why was starting to deeply anchor me into being a present and a wholehearted mother, wife, worker, friend, and family member. My why was to be the same person day and night. As Kari Schwear of GrayTonic succinctly states, "Your why has to be of deep value. It cannot be a wishy-washy desire. It also cannot be because your spouse or someone else thinks you should. This is about YOU and only you."[4]

Even though my why was firmly planted, I still had this nagging fear lurking in the back of my mind asking, *Do I want to do this forever*? The fears I faced were very similar to when I got my first road bike. I was exhilarated by the speed of being clipped into my road bike, yet at the same time, I was terrified that I would not be able to clip out quickly enough to stop at a stop sign or stoplight. It sounds silly, but at the beginning of riding my road bike, I would only go down roads where I could make right turns so I could continue on my ride and not need to make urgent stops. As you can imagine, this limited where I could ride my bicycle. The fear of falling literally gripped me every time I stepped onto the bike. *What if I cannot stop and unclip? What if I hit a car? What if I fall?* The "what ifs" raced through my mind, even though at the same time I loved riding my new road bike.

Taking the first step to stop drinking when you never hit a rock bottom can feel much like this: *What if I tell others I have quit, but then I decide to go back? What if—*

The what ifs are strong when you embark on an alcohol-free journey.

"What if I don't really have a problem?" is a big question for gray area drinkers on their alcohol-free journey, when the temptations of alcohol feel much like a joker, playing pranks on your mind, convincing you you've got this. This is particularly hard when the ones closest to you never thought you had a problem. Alcohol is so ingrained into every part of our society that choosing to abstain from it or saying "I can drink if I want to, but I choose not to" makes those around us question their own relationship with alcohol.

ꟹ

Slowly, I started practicing stopping and starting on my bike, easing into the feeling of clipping and unclipping. Getting used to this feeling, falling only once or twice, I finally started to let go of my fears and trust myself. This opened up all kinds of new rides for me. It no longer had a grip on me; my fear of falling or crashing had dissipated. Slowly, alcohol was starting to lose its grip on me as well. The increase in energy starts to empower you. The feeling of being fog-free is exhilarating, just like the road bike was for me.

I started to enjoy waking up early. Now I love my mornings, feeling great when I open my eyes, replete with a surge of energy to take on the day. Waking up without a dry mouth or upset stomach or a cloudy mind never gets old. I pop out of bed now, when I used to barely be able to open one eye. I have learned to fill my bucket first . . . before the day and the world take from it.

Just like on my new road bike, I was beginning to feel better and wanted to see where this new ride would take me now that I was learning how to clip into being alcohol-free. Even though physically I was starting to feel better, I still was not sure I wanted to break up with alcohol forever. Was it possible to go back to where I could take it or leave it once again? I started looking into podcasts, books, and even asking my Sober Sisters if they knew of any successful "moderators" (individuals who were every-now-again drinkers) so I could learn their tricks.

The Infamous Pitcher Plant

I reached out to Stacy, an interior decorator with three children, with whom I had bonded over the reset. Stacy and I had similar type A personalities, go-getters who were both under the illusion that alcohol was the solution to calm our rat race. Married to a highly successful salesman, Stacy understood the pressure I was under at work to hit sales goals and the party life that came along with it. An instant friendship was born.

Stacy and I started taking on more of a leadership role within our Sober Sis group, as we were outspoken and regularly posted on Marco Polo. However, even though I was doing "the work"—listening to podcasts, reading "quit lit" books, talking to my new therapist, and journaling—the relentless alcohol jokester kept appearing, playing tricks on my mind, asking, *What if we could just drink on occasion*?

I couldn't find any individuals who were successfully "moderating" their alcohol intake, online or in any books or podcasts, so I jumped on Marco Polo and asked Stacy what her thoughts were on moderation. Stacy quickly replied, "No, take it from me, this is my second time doing the Sober Sis 21-Day Reset. I quit drinking for six months after doing this reset a while back and figured I had regained control of my relationship with alcohol. Over time, I allowed myself one or two drinks here or there at social functions. Slowly but surely over the next year, I was back to my gray area drinking again."

Even though a good amount of time had lapsed for Stacy, the alcohol trap had swallowed her back into its distortions and deceit. I trusted Stacy and valued her opinions and insights on this journey. Her story left me fearful of going through the dreadful first thirty days of detoxing again, only to fall right back to where I had worked so hard to escape. Now over thirty days alcohol-free, I felt the best physically that I had felt in a long time, and I began to ask myself, *Did I want to go back to that place? Was it even worth it?*

By believing we can control our alcohol, we circle the lid of the infamous pitcher plant. The pitcher plant has a pitcher-shaped leaf with a long tubular opening. It is a pitfall trap for insects who land on its rim seeking the sweet nectar and falling further and further down into its deep cavity. Like a fly who feeds on the sweet nectar of the pitcher plant, we too circle the rim of the bottle, inching our way down into the trap.

Our cravings intensify over time, our tolerance of alcohol grows, and only when we decide to quit drinking do we even realize we are in the pitcher plant.

It was becoming clear that each of us had been lured down into the pitcher plant's sweet nectar by a traumatic event in our lives. But as we were slipping down its deep cavity, we were oblivious to our entrapment as it is leisurely and insidious. The fly doesn't flee the pitcher plant because it cannot see the danger. We, too, can not see that we are slipping down alcohol's steep chamber of deceit.

Author William Porter shared another analogy on a Zoom call with our Sober Sis group, in which he clearly illustrated why we cannot control our alcohol:

> Imagine driving on a road at thirty mph where you must maintain that speed. You cannot go faster nor slower—just keeping at thirty mph. You've got your foot down on the accelerator at a specific amount to keep your speed at thirty miles per hour. For a good bit, you stay at a steady pace of thirty mph on the road, but then the road ends into wet mud and grass. This slows the vehicle down, but you still have to maintain that thirty mph, which is nearly impossible to do because you have to press harder on the accelerator to get back up to thirty mph. The problem is when the mud and wet grass ends, you go back out onto concrete, where you fly out of control. Trying to control your alcohol is much like this over time.[5]

For a while, controlling our alcohol works on the smooth road, staying steady at thirty mph, then something changes (your tolerance) and you veer off the smooth road onto rough terrain, where maintaining thirty mph is challenging given the unpredictable landscape. Gradually, the "relaxing" feeling we get with alcohol requires more and more alcohol over time, chasing that same effect.

Just like the fly, we unknowingly fall deeper into the infamous pitcher plant's tubular trap convincing ourselves we are in control of our alcohol when in all actuality it controls us.

The Veil Drops

While reading *This Naked Mind* by Annie Grace, I could feel the veil slowly being lifted off my eyes when I learned that alcohol is ethanol. Ethanol is made from distillation of fermented starch. It is a good solvent, creates other chemicals, and can be mixed with gasoline.

Annie says in her book, "The most glaring truth about alcohol is that it is ethanol. As in, we are drinking the same substance we put in our gas tank."[6]

The old saying "Once you know, you can never not know" rang true for me as I continued reading Annie's bold truths about alcohol. The sheer fact that most of us must mix alcohol with a mixer, just to make it palatable, should give us pause.

Annie also says, "Alcohol scored as the most harmful drug, with an overall harm score of seventy-two. Heroin came in second with a harm score of fifty-five and crack cocaine scored third with a score of fifty-four."[7]

I was stunned. The first question that came to my mind was *Why wasn't I warned of this danger*? The other thing that is so disconcerting is that we get so many warnings about nicotine and meth but hardly any about the dangers of alcohol.

It has been said that if alcohol were discovered today, it would never be approved for usage, as it is a known carcinogen. Annie goes on to say, "The International Agency for Research on Cancer (IARC) declared alcohol a carcinogen in 1988. Alcohol itself, ethanol, is a known carcinogen and alcoholic beverages can contain at least fifteen other carcinogenic compounds including arsenic, formaldehyde, and lead."[8]

As the days progressed, my curiosity grew as to why I was going along with the herd when it clearly was not working in my life. I started asking myself new questions like *Why do I want to drink ethanol when I am choosing healthy options the rest of the day? Why are we normalizing this highly addictive drug? Why do we think we can control it? Why do we believe the lies society tells us about it? If it is a carcinogenic like the American Cancer Society*[9] *says it is, why are we all celebrating it and encouraging each other to drink more of it? Why aren't we discussing the dangers of it? Why are we making each other feel shame and guilt for being addicted to it, when it is more addictive than nicotine and methamphetamine?*

And most importantly, when we say "Alcohol is no longer serving me," my question is: When *was* it serving you?

We need to ask ourselves: What *do* we believe alcohol is providing or adding to our lives?

My mind was consumed with answering all these questions. I had ample driving time in the car to my sales appointments, so I took full advantage of listening to all kinds of podcasts on drinking. After listening to some of them, I would jump online with my Sober Sis group, saying, "Hey, it's Meg again. I have been listening to Rachel Hart's podcasts on why we drink and what is driving our drinking behaviors. Just as it was recommended in our daily emails in Sober Sis, I highly recommend listening to this podcast." I became the "podcast reporter" in our Marco Polo group: *Reporting live from Delaware . . . you need to listen to the "Does Alcohol Solve an Emotion?" episode on Rachel Hart's* Take a Break from Drinking *podcast*! Over time, my online sobriety group began to lean on me for where to go to learn more about how alcohol was impacting our minds, our bodies, and our spirits.

Something was also shifting in my brain as I continued to educate myself on the truths about alcohol. I could see that time and space without this substance combined with the education on the truths about it was slowly retraining and rewiring my brain on how

I viewed it. Even though many of us weren't sure if we would be alcohol-free forever, I got online and made a sort of declaration post:

> I am realizing I don't want to count the days anymore. This is not a willpower thing but rather an understanding to want to change my mindset and view of alcohol. I am never going to view alcohol the same way again. I want to understand why I am drinking in the first place. At first, I thought I was just going to take a break from alcohol, but now, after listening to these podcasts and doing this reset, I am not so sure. I told my husband that I am not sure this is a forever thing, but I feel so much better. I am more present with my kids and at work, so I want to explore this even more. Every time in the past when I have tried to stop drinking, it was sheer willpower and never lasted more than two weeks. Now I am understanding why I am drinking and why I want to stop. I am learning how to choose differently and not give into my habitual wine at night.

Instead of sheer willpower to not drink like I had experienced in the past with cleanses and diets, this time was different. Yes, the detoxing period took some willpower, but it was different this time around. It was defogging my gray lens, helping me understand why I was choosing alcohol, and awakening me to its lies, illusions, and myths. I had truly believed it provided so many things to me, when in all actuality it did just the opposite. I was starting to see the trap I had fallen into and that I had the choice to stay in it or work my way out of it. I started to become more curious about the idea of never drinking again.

In addition to feeling better, I was starting to see a change in my outward appearance as well. My entire life, I have struggled with eczema and dry, sensitive skin. Now my rashes and skin were clearing up, plus my eyes were also becoming brighter. I noticed the puffiness in my face was decreasing. The stomach problems I had grown accustomed to were no longer an issue. It dawned on me that I had never heard someone who is drinking say, "Alcohol has given me this, that, or any kind of improvement in my life." Now improvements were slowly appearing, giving me more reasons to stay on the alcohol-free path.

Even though outward improvements were occurring, every time I heard the word "alcohol" or "drinking" it felt like a sharp knife poking at an open wound. When I would hear songs on the radio about alcohol, I had to switch the station . . . a *lot*! I wanted and needed to rewire my brain with the right messages, no longer allowing subliminal seductive lies about alcohol to sing in my ears. I was becoming keenly aware of all the places that pro-drinking messages were being subliminally embedded into my subconscious as I was ingesting its toxic deceptions. I changed my radio station settings, I changed whom I followed on social media, and I started following sobriety sites. Slowly, over time, my mind was being rewired with healthier messages.

Upon completion of our 21-Day Reset, with an additional month of being alcohol-free behind us, ten of the thirty of us decided to break off into a totally alcohol-free group for an additional ninety days, and we signed up for the Alcohol-Free Lifestyle (AFL) Course with Sober Sis. The ten of us wanted to know what it felt like to be over one hundred days alcohol-free.

It was here in our intimate group of ten that we dove deeper into the possibility of doing this forever. Our common thread was suffering, and each of us was diving deeper into what initially drove us to drink. The irony of us trying to control our alcohol and the idea of control in our lives allowed me to see how these two old beliefs were working in tandem, keeping me trapped in gray area drinking.

It was becoming more evident that controlling my alcohol was going to be very difficult, much like trying to control many other things in my life.

The Lie: "I Can Control My Drinking"

The Truth: Most gray area drinkers want desperately to go back to being an occasional drinker. Still under the illusion that we can control our drinking, many of us try moderation, realizing it takes an enormous amount of effort and self-awareness to keep tabs on our drinking. The amount of effort to keep within the guard rails of moderation usually results in sheer willpower that wanes over time, resulting in going back to our old drinking patterns. By trying to control our alcohol, we circle the rim of the infamous pitcher plant, where unknowingly we can be lured back to its sweet nectar and trapped once again. There is no freedom in that.

Did You Know?

According to the National Institute on Alcohol Abuse and Alcoholism, "It is common for people to consume alcohol in an effort to cope with stress, sleep disturbances, and even boredom. Beginning in adolescence, females are more likely to suffer from anxiety disorders and depression, increasing the motivation to drink alcohol for temporary relief. Unfortunately, this approach tends to make problems worse, not better, and increases the risk for AUD (alcohol use disorder) and other adverse consequences. Although alcohol temporarily dampens the body's response to stress, feelings of stress and anxiety not only return but worsen once the alcohol wears off. Over time, alcohol misuse can cause adaptations in the brain that intensify the stress response. As a result, drinking alcohol to cope amplifies feelings of stress, anxiety, and depression, and one may end up drinking to fix problems caused by the alcohol itself."[10]

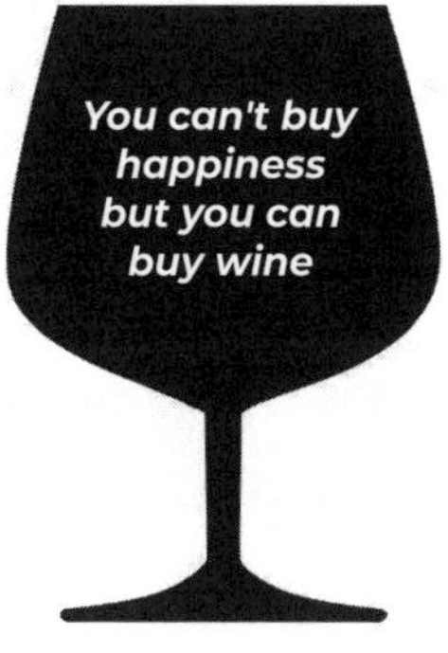

CHAPTER FOUR

"BEING SOBER IS BORING!"

I had always loved entertaining, but entertaining while newly sober was different and a vast departure from my typical party-planning routine. For most of my life, alcohol was at the center of my social world. It was the defining feature of what I thought was fun, what I thought was a good time. Entertaining is something my husband and I love to do, always making sure everyone is having the best time possible. But I was emotionally raw and sensitive and wasn't sure how things would go entertaining alcohol-free.

We were throwing our annual Christmas party, and our guests were expected at our house by 4 p.m. I had set up a mocktail bar full of lots of fun nonalcoholic drinks and nonalcoholic beers. I also stocked a full bar for those who wanted to drink. Being around others who were drinking didn't really bother me. I had long kept alcohol in the house without a thought of getting into it. What really scared me was *Would I be any fun without it?* That old, conditioned belief that I could only be fun or have fun with alcohol was now being put to the test.

But I had a plan.

My mocktails awaited me, the house was decorated, and the food was prepared. I was excited and nervous about how the night might unfold, just staying focused on actually being fully present for these holidays.

As we sat down to eat Christmas dinner, I noticed that one of my guests was now a full bottle into her favorite chardonnay. This was the first time that both my sister and I were not drinking in the presence of this guest. In the past, alcohol always made the uncomfortable silence or awkwardness of social interactions disappear. Now this uncomfortable silence was staring me right in the face during our Christmas meal. As we passed around the honey-baked ham and my aunt's famous spinach casserole, you could feel the tension at the table. Getting used to the uncomfortable was a new frontier for me, and I was just trying to ignore its presence. Then, out of nowhere, like a blade slicing through the thick tension, this guest said the unthinkable, stating in a joking manner (but it certainly was not, to say the least) that my sister and I were "boring."

All I could hear was "*You* are boring."

As these words came out of her mouth, they cut through me like the sharpest knife she could throw at my biggest fear in getting sober. The wine witch suddenly reappeared, flying around the dining room table as if she knew this moment would come, laughing hysterically in my face: *See, my little pretty? I told you—you would be boring without the alcohol. Hee-hee-hee!*

My raw feelings recoiled at the words spoken at the table. I had to get up to regain my composure. I walked outside to take out the trash and took several deep breaths. *Is this really happening?* I wondered. *Is this really true?*

My mind raced with doubts as a big craving washed over me, urging me to just give in and say *f*ck it.* Facing uncharted waters where I would normally drink to quell my nerves was no longer an option, and now, coupled with my guest's harsh comment, all I wanted to do was grab a drink to numb out even more. I had to stand in this horrible feeling and let it pass. I knew that if I gave in and had a drink, it would solve nothing. I had to see it for what it really was—it was not about me; it was more of a fear *she* had about not drinking.

After taking several deep breaths of the night's cold, refreshing air, I came to the realization that she, too, had fallen prey to the old, conditioned thought that the only way you can have fun is with a drink.

After the party, I connected with my online Sober Sisters, who quickly swooped in to pick me back up. Still the pain remained, but the connection with these ladies who deeply understood that same fear of no longer being fun was what carried me through that night. All the women in the group chimed in with the truth that being hungover all day is what's *really* boring. And that not playing with my kids because I was too tired from drinking the night before is boring too. Boring because I was too much in an alcohol-induced fog to truly listen to what others were saying at a party. The truth is, I am no longer boring, because I am present and not numbing out the good and the bad.

The following year, this same guest came again for our annual Christmas party. Now I cared more about how I felt and less how others felt, fully enjoying every moment of my annual Christmas party. At the end of the dinner, our infamous guest enthused, "This was really fun. Thanks for having me!"

First Feels

Over the next several months, I gradually shed who I used to be, someone who was the life of the party. The beach was a big drinking destination for my husband and me, where as soon as we parked the car, we never got back in it. That way, we could bar hop all over our small beach town. Now, driving into town, I looked at each bar and restaurant with trepidation, feeling like our old stomping grounds were a new foreign land to navigate alcohol-free. As I started to unpack, I debated about ordering takeout, not wanting to face the memories of my old drinking days. I knew I would have to face these memories at some point. Besides, takeout sushi isn't the same as eating it in our favorite restaurant. For years, when we would frequent that restaurant, I would sit at the bar sipping on my favorite prosecco, chatting up the bartenders while I noshed on my sushi.

I conjured up the courage and decided to head out. As I approached the restaurant's door, I was sweating. My cold, clammy hands were trembling a tad bit because this was my first time-out since I ditched the drink. *Can I do this?* I wondered for the umpteenth time. I sat at the bar with fear of judgment and bewilderment at what the bartender would say. I timidly asked, "What kind of mocktails do you have?"

He responded, "Do you like fruity or a more sour taste?"

Hmm, what a good question.

I didn't know.

I responded, "I like a refreshing taste like grapefruit."

"Great! I know just what to make you!" he replied.

Whew, I thought, *thank God, because I have no clue.*

A sense of relief and excitement for my new drink washed over me. When my beautiful zero-proof drink arrived at the bar, I felt like I fit in. I knew my awkwardness was mostly in my head, so

I settled in on the barstool and began to sip on my drink, which was refreshing and delicious. There I was, eating my favorite sushi, sipping on a cool mocktail. My first win all alone. A new sense of pride burst from deep within. *This isn't as scary as I thought,* I mused. *I can still have fun, wake up refreshed, and be able to enjoy all the beach had to offer.*

Even though I had my first win under my belt, my first sales meeting proved to be a much bigger challenge. Our sales meetings normally revolved around a lot of alcohol, which left me fearful and questioning my strength on this journey. My coworkers knew me as a confident leader on the team who was always up for a fun time at meetings. Fear of what my manager may think also took hold of my thoughts. I would have to face a happy hour and a long steak house dinner where the wine would be endlessly flowing.

As I got to the hotel, my phone blew up about happy hour at the hotel lobby before we were to head out to the restaurant. I knew this was going to be a challenge. I reached out for connection first, giving my Sober Sisters my plan for the evening. I asked them to be on hand if I got too weak, to hold me accountable to stay on the alcohol-free path. I decided to read some of my quit lit book, *We Are the Luckiest* by Laura McKowen, arriving late to happy hour as a result. I volunteered to be the designated driver to dinner from the hotel, knowing that this would relieve me of some of the "drinking expectation" throughout the night. I survived happy hour, and since I was late, it was only happy *half* hour for me. We all piled into my car and headed to the steak house.

As we sat down for dinner, the same uneasy feeling of awkwardness came flooding into my body . . . that God-awful anxiety that I always quelled with a drink. The waiter came around the table and asked, "Red or white wine?"

Like this is your only choice. Like it is a given that you will drink, right?

I asked the waiter if he had any nonalcoholic beers. This is an always interesting question to this day when I go out to eat. The waiter has to think for a minute—do they even have non-alcoholic beer on hand? Every time this happens, it feels as if the music screeches in the restaurant and everyone is looking at you with eyes that scream, *Wait, you're not going to drink alcohol? What is wrong with you*?!

The waiter told me he had to check to see if they had any non-alcoholic beer.

"Great, thanks," I quietly responded, trying not to bring any more attention to my non-alcoholic request when it felt like the entire room was staring at me.

My frosty mug full of nonalcoholic beer arrived at the table with what looked like real beer chilling in it. In my mind, those across the table who could not hear my order looked relieved. Their faces said, *Oh good, she* is *drinking with us.*

Looking back, I know much of this is how I perceived things, not how they were, but when it is your first experience going against the grain in the masses, you feel like you are naked in a room of people wondering what is going on with you. It was another lie I had believed: *if everyone's doing it, it can't be that bad.*

It did not stop the inquiring minds of a few who sat near me when they heard a non-alcoholic request. It is always interesting how many questions folks will have about someone not drinking. "Are you on a diet? Are you doing a cleanse?" a few asked. Why anyone cares whether or not I drink is a new awareness that had not even entered my realm of thinking. I simply said, "No, I am not drinking."

I left it at that, not really giving anyone any further explanation. Why do we need to explain why we are not drinking? Why is the only socially acceptable answer is that we're doing a cleanse or on a diet? We feel pressured to reassure others: *Don't worry, this isn't forever, this is just a temporary pause*! Is it that when we say we aren't drinking, others feel that same small, quiet voice within them questioning why *they* drink?

I thought I was in the clear, but then my manager leans over and pushes it further. I decide to tell him I quit drinking because it was no longer serving me. Period. He looks surprised and then says, "Good for you." I think to myself, *Yes, good for me. Good for me for surviving this alcohol-filled, "judgy" dinner.*

After guzzling multiple bottles of wine at dinner, my entire work crew headed back to the hotel for even more ethanol at the hotel bar once again. I made a brief appearance at the bar, sweating under my top. Full of anxiety, counting the minutes till I could make a mad dash for my hotel room, I make the rounds at the bar. My mind races with thoughts: *Can I make it? Can I act like mingling at the bar is not the hardest feat bestowed upon me*? This is where, before committing to stay alcohol-free, I would have continued to drink to subdue my social anxiety with my coworkers. Now that was no longer an option. That option was simply not there for me.

Instead, a sweaty, clammy, anxiety-filled version of myself was navigating how to make an appearance at the bar and get the hell out of Dodge. I had to keep my brave, smiling face on display, chatting like all is fine in the world. My anxiety is pressing against my skin, pleading with me and my brain to be dealt with. I realize I am worn out from the night, and I am hitting a wall. I quietly disappear from the bar like a Houdini act. Another big win.

I get on Marco Polo with my Sober Sisters and tell them I *did* it. I share the insecurities I had with facing all my peers without alcohol. I discussed how hard it was, how awkward it felt to sit in it, and how brave it is to go against the grain. All my life I followed what everyone else thought was acceptable and popular, and now, for the first time, I was putting myself first. A new sense of self-worth was blooming slowly within me.

The next day, I woke up feeling great as my coworkers sluggishly dragged themselves to breakfast. At breakfast, I was questioned about my disappearance from the bar last night. Where did I go? Why did I leave? Again, who cares? But when alcohol is the main contestant at the show, and you abandon ship, everyone wants to know why. In their defense, my coworkers were used to me being the last one at the bar. The old me would have been gallivanting around with her drink in hand. I tell them honestly, simply, that I was tired and wanted to go to bed.

I survived my first sales meeting with a new sense of pride that I can do this and next time it will be easier.

Boring in the Bedroom

It has been a "brutiful" journey, as author of *Carry On, Warrior*, Glennon Doyle, says—both beautiful and brutal[1]—an amazing transformational experience of feeling the pain, healing it, and ultimately seeing the beauty in it.

My husband, Paul, and I enjoyed drinking when we met in our late twenties. We both loved to entertain and throw a good party, which always included lots of alcohol. When we married, this love of hosting parties at our house continued even after we had kids. Much of our connection time was built around drinking.

When I quit drinking, Paul joined me in being alcohol-free, which was an enormous amount of support on my journey. But his journey was very different from mine. He could switch his drinking on and off easily. Take or leave it. Me, not so much. I had to dive into the inner work of why I was using alcohol as a crutch. For most of the women in my Sober Sis group, their husbands continued to drink during their journey.

Stacy describes what it was like having her adult children and husband drinking on her journey:

> It was not only my family who was drinking, but it was also our closest friends, and we bought a cottage in the middle of what they call the "Texas wine trail." Alcohol was all around me, all the time. I was at a point where I realized it did not have to do with anyone else, it was just about me. Nobody could help me do it. It had to be my own journey. It had to be separate from what my husband was doing; I had to stay in my own lane and only worry about myself and not anybody else. There were a lot of moments where I had to rely on our sober group to help me get through it because everyone around me was drinking. It is a lot like eating habits—if you have forty pounds to lose and your spouse doesn't, you get to a point where you're going to take care of yourself and do what you need to do to lose the weight, or you are not. It has nothing to do with the other people around you. They can't lose the weight for you. You have to do it yourself. It was the same thing with drinking. My husband was supportive of what I was doing, but he didn't really get it. I got to a space where it didn't matter what he thought.

> The most challenging part was not drinking and being around people who I could see were being affected by the alcohol. It was a really good self-check to see things that I didn't see before. And, for me, the biggest part that came out of that was I got to know myself so well, and it ended it up being a highlight to what I believed I deserved. I think the biggest result of not drinking was the work I had to do on myself so I could be content without alcohol in my life.
>
> This journey has to be just for you, and you need to be ready to do it just for yourself. Doesn't matter what others think, what matters is what you think. A big piece in this alcohol-free journey is taking full accountability for yourself, your own life, your own feelings. There is no one else to blame. It doesn't work to say, "I can't do this because my spouse is still drinking." My why comes from deep within me and has nothing to do with what's going on around me.

Even though my husband and I were on the same journey, being alcohol-free makes you more aware of your surroundings, like Stacy says. Things that I was too fogged out to see were now crystal clear and would get under my skin in our marriage. I found myself easily irritated with many people. The judgmental side of me was now at the surface. When we judge others, it gives us the quick dopamine hit that we are okay and don't need fixing; it's the other person who needs help. *Au contraire*! I started examining my judgment and could see where most of my life, I was the person trying to be perfect, to not *be* judged, only giving my judgment to others. It was a shift from judgment to curiosity. Getting curious about others' lenses, experiences, and how they viewed the world allowed me to stay open to love and move away from judgment.

This realization and deep dive into my inner work gave way to me showing up differently. Whereas I used to sit with Paul drinking the night away, now I was pouring not into my glass but into myself. I needed him to know that the immense amount of time I was doing the inner work on myself had nothing to do with not loving him. Just the opposite was true. I was learning to heal the triggers and old habitual patterns of reaction I had suppressed for years with a glass of wine.

As we were shifting out of drinking together and going to bed earlier, I was waking up earlier, which resulted in less affection in the bedroom. As a focal point in our marriage, alcohol usually led to me being tipsy and then, of course, more inebriated in the bedroom. Now that was gone. Instead, I felt like a big awkward elephant was sitting on our bed at night. What was once not discussed because it happened frequently when we were inebriated was now creating more tension between us. I was so tired at night, leaving such little bandwidth for the bedroom. This was a major change for Paul, who wasn't used to me this way.

For the first time in our marriage, we started to argue repeatedly. We decided to go to an online marriage counselor to help us move through this shift. We had many productive sessions with our marriage counselor, learning how our childhood and past were impacting how we were showing up and reacting to each other. This was incredibly helpful. By taking alcohol out of the equation, we found we had more clarity and compassion toward one another as we revealed why we were showing up the way we were.

In the bedroom, we had to unlearn and learn new ways of coming together. For some, being sober in the bedroom was better because they could remember it all. For me, it was just the opposite. I felt like alcohol had corroded not only the wire to my inner knowing but also my intimacy wire. It felt like wires were trying to reconnect to new outlets, grappling for a spark of connection in a brand-new way.

During one of the online sessions with our marriage counselor, we discussed our intimacy issues. She purposefully looked at me and said, "Meg, I am going to need you to go green when you are on yellow with sex."

I just stared at her, dumbfounded. The little girl within me jumped up and said, *Is she telling me just to be submissive*? *Just deny your body's physical changes and give in*? More importantly, my inner knowing was screaming back, *She is telling me to abandon myself just to please my husband in the bedroom*!

Needless to say, that was our last session with that marriage counselor. Instead, I sat down with Paul, discussing how I wanted to be intimate not because I felt like I had to but because I *wanted* to and could therefore enjoy it. I explained that all systems were shutting down earlier in the evenings, and I let him know that I was going to honor my body, mind, and spirit over going "green."

I was no longer willing to abandon myself to please even my own husband. Paul is always so understanding and supportive, so we adjusted and shifted into another new routine of going to bed earlier together. It took some time, but my mind and body began to heal, allowing for these wires of intimacy to reconnect once again in the evenings. This shift was the slowest one on my journey. As Glennon Doyle says, "Every time you're given a choice between disappointing someone else and disappointing yourself, your duty is to disappoint that someone else. Your job throughout your entire life is to disappoint as many people as it takes to avoid disappointing yourself."[2]

I was finally waking up to no longer disappointing and abandoning myself, now always choosing what felt true and good to me. Choosing myself over and over again began to appear in many facets of my life throughout my alcohol-free journey, each time like a test to see if I would choose my needs, my beliefs, my voice, and my preferences over external validation. These choices arise, asking you to choose only the ones that bring you joy and forego the ones that don't. The beauty is that every day we get to make a choice, asking ourselves: *Will you reconnect with your one true self, or will you abandon her to please everyone else?*

Knowing Ourselves

As we were teasing out what drove us to drink, our Sober Sis AFL group began working through the Enneagram, a system of nine personality types that allow us to take a deeper dive into self-awareness, gaining knowledge of our inner selves.

"The power of the Enneagram map lies in its highly accurate articulation of the automatic patterns associated with the personalities it describes," Beatrice Chestnut writes in her book *The Complete Enneagram.*[3] Upon completion of the Enneagram test, my results revealed almost a tie (no shocker) between a number two (The Helper, a.k.a. The Rescuer) and number one (The Reformer, a.k.a. The Perfectionist). But it was apparent that my defaulting to old patterns could become a strength if I continued to do the inner work to heal them. The Enneagram helped me see how I viewed the world, what my motivations to do things were, and what sparked my fears. The Enneagram gives us the compassion not only for ourselves but also for our loved ones and how their Enneagram personality type views the world.

The Enneagram teaches us how to take our vices and turn them into virtues. When we do this, we transform into our "true" higher selves. For example, The Perfectionist gets things done and is task oriented, but when we relinquish the high standards we put on ourselves as perfectionists, we number ones can get things done without the added pressure of perfectionism.

When a number two, The Helper, goes into helping without wanting anything in return and works on seeing her own needs, only then is she in her higher self-mode. The healthy number two only helps when asked and wants to—not because she feels like she has to—resulting in a truly altruistic higher self. I could now vividly see how the "old me" was showing up in reactions to life's challenges with a desire to control, fix, and rescue . . . and to do it all perfectly.

Before doing this Enneagram and inner work, I didn't realize that I was a highly sensitive person. Other people's energies engulfed my own. I could easily perceive and read people's moods and needs, always leaving me feeling like I needed to help them. The people pleaser and rescuer in me would jump into action, like the time when my sister's son was having trouble breathing and the doctors had discovered some nodules on his lungs. I sprang into action. *I have to help him*! *I have to help her figure out this diagnosis as to what is going on—I have to take care of them*!

Without any consideration, I called many of the physicians I knew at work for a second and third opinion as to what was going on with my nephew. I worried about him and my sister. I researched all the possible things these unknown nodules could be. Like a rat who has been trained to run the maze to get the treat, I sprang into rescue mode, zipping through the maze, running into walls, but continuing to forge onward. I had several hypotheses on what was happening with my nephew based on my doctor's assessments, and I needed to rescue him immediately.

When I did not hear back from my sister right away, I was panic stricken. My husband looked at me and asked, "Did she ask for your help?" It was like a slap across my face. He was right: she hadn't even *asked* for my help. I was just doing what I always do, what I felt I had to do. *Who I used to be was glaring starkly back at me.* The Enneagram allowed me to see with compassion I was in autopilot mode. Now, with alcohol out of the picture, the unearthing and revelation of who I used to be started to give way to the "true me."

The Unbecoming and Becoming

When I was drinking, I would always ask my sister, "Are you mad at me?" The chronic people pleaser in me was constantly paranoid that I was disappointing others around me. In my mind, I was never enough, *it* was never enough: I could never make everyone happy. I just thought if my little engine worked harder, it would arrive at its destination—complete approval. *I think I can—I think I can—I think I can.* After I was alcohol-free for some time, my sister said, "You know, you don't ask me anymore if I am mad at you. You used to ask me so often that it started to make me wonder if I was doing something to upset you; it was confusing."

I hadn't even realized I was doing this in the past until she brought it to my attention. I didn't even realize I had so many insecurities that I needed constant reassurance from the closest people in my life. I was always looking outside myself, over and over again, for approval.

During this time, the unbecoming and undoing of decades of avoidance left me at times with very little emotional bandwidth. I was happy, on top of the world, one moment and overwhelmed with emotion the next. This time period made me want to crawl into a cocoon and hide from the world, but I knew it was time to stop hiding and live like God intended me to do. Feelings carry messages, and when we numb them, we miss the lessons they hold for us. The alcohol-free journey was a process of stripping off all my old beliefs and growing new skin, new beliefs, which were beginning to strengthen that very important voice within.

Feeling all these feelings for the first time is like a newborn learning to walk. You may fall, but you keep trying. You get up holding onto the side of the couch for support with each new fumbling step. Each attempt wears you out. This is why newborns take lots of naps. They are feeling, absorbing, taking on all new things—it's exhausting. My mantra during this alcohol-free journey is *Be gentle with yourself.* As adults, feeling these feelings for the first time are just as exhausting, but there is no time for a nap. *Be gentle with yourself; it's exhausting.*

Dr. Brené Brown has a great segment entitled "Brené on FFTs" on her *Unlocking Us* podcast where she describes FFTs (F*cking First Times) as a strategy. She describes how naming our FFTs and owning our hard things gives us power to effect change and instill purpose. Some first times could be the first Christmas, wedding, or birthday party you attend alcohol-free.

Dr. Brown describes how being new at something or trying a new thing makes us incredibly vulnerable. The awkward, uncomfortable time comes right after the excitement of trying something new. Being new at something is the epitome of vulnerability. She goes on to say that the only way to get to the other side is to get through the hard middle part.[4]

Many times, we don't try something new because we are too afraid to be vulnerable, so we stay where we are comfortable. If we don't know how to do it well and have some expertise, we don't do it.

The firsts are the hardest and extend sometimes past the first year of being alcohol-free. Feeling things that had been dulled by alcohol for years now felt intensely sharp, poignant, and awkward. Most of us haven't felt these feelings in a long time—sometimes years—because we've been numbing them with food, alcohol, sex, shopping, or whatever your thing is. To me, this was the hardest part of the alcohol-free journey. Early on in my journey, my new, raw skin allowed these feelings to get under my flesh because there was so little protection. I felt barren, naked, and exposed to whatever came my way as this new transformation was occurring. I was easily angered and overly sensitive to comments. In fact, I was defensive and hypersensitive to everything around me.

Shedding my old skin took time. Learning to grow in places you have suppressed and escaped for years take patience, but it yields a new you that glows with peace and clarity. I could feel, inside each win, a building of my muscle of being okay with being in the minority, knowing that I was for the first time listening to my needs and awakening to the old, programmed beliefs. The becoming means sitting with these feelings, acknowledging them, honoring them, and then letting them go. It is not about changing who you are. Your feelings, pain, and emotions are there to teach you. They'll teach you a spiritual lesson if you will allow it.

As a society, we are not taught to sit with our emotions. Sitting with our emotions can be difficult; the enormity of them can be engulfing at times, but this is where we grow strong, ladies. Our emotions do *not* define us. The courage to sit with them, honor them, and release them through journaling, movement, meditation, or just venting them out in community helps us move through them. The ability to surrender and accept what is builds our courage, tenacity, and perseverance. This is how we reconnect to our heart, soul, and spirit.

After some time, you will see that when these feelings arise for the second, third, and fourth time around, they will come on with less intensity and more like an old friend you keep running into. Like building a muscle, we need to exercise feeling our feelings over and over, letting go over and over, until we are strong enough to know this too shall pass and that small, consistent wins are what create lasting change.

The unbecoming phase is also the unraveling of your limiting beliefs, roles that no longer serve you, and, most importantly, prioritizing your needs and wants. What does unbecoming look like? No longer are you the inebriated wife who, after a few drinks, is ready to get it on. You no longer are the friend who wants to stay up to the wee hours drinking the night away and forgetting most of the conversation. But on the bright side, you are the mother who wakes up fully present for your children. You are the mother who has energy to take them to the park and play with them. You are the wife who is more engaged and present in conversations with her partner. You are the consummate professional who is more astute at work. The friend who is fully present and authentically connecting in conversations.

However, it can still feel isolating at times when those around you don't understand your new ways or only know you in the old way. Be gentle with yourself as the true you is showing up for all the loved ones surrounding you who may not know who you are quite yet. It takes time. It takes time to learn your vulnerabilities, your unhealed wounds and trauma, but navigating the uncharted land comes with finding the beauty in the mess.

By examining my inner child in therapy, I could see parts of the little girl who thought she needed alcohol to fit in. The little girl who desperately wanted to be accepted and be enough. The adolescent who bought into the societal message that alcohol was the solution, the young woman who used it as a crutch, and the mother who used it to navigate stressful situations. Now, without a substance to numb you, the rough edges of your past beckon for you to deal with them. You rub up against them, they *hurt*, and you're not sure how to react and handle all these new feelings.

These pointy edges are pointing you to freedom. It is hard to lean into the edges that were softened by alcohol. But alcohol-free, you slowly begin to see they are there to guide you. As Jenn Kautsch says, "Alcohol used to soften your edges; now, alcohol-free, you get your edge back!"[5]

As I was gaining strength with my wins, I was now ready to tell my closest friends about my alcohol-free journey. I wanted it to be a private conversation with each of them rather than during a social event together. Each time I was on the phone with a friend explaining that I had quit drinking, my hands would slightly tremble, and my heart would race with the uncertainty of how they would react. Would they still want to hang out? Would we still be friends? Would they still invite me to parties? The little girl who was ostracized in fifth grade poked her head out in fear. The eighth grader who felt alcohol helped her fit in with her friends was left wondering, *Would there be anyone left to hang out with?* Each phone call was building a new sense of who I was becoming and what I stood for. Each conversation was an explanation as to why I had chosen to quit drinking and a testament of going against the grain of society.

I realized that putting yourself first is the very way you learn to stop pleasing people and learn how to love yourself more. It is an act of self-validation versus external validation. I was also making myself more accountable by sharing my journey—making my future successes more likely. I was setting an example for my friends to begin pondering their relationship with alcohol as well. By sharing our truths on our alcohol-free journey, we also destigmatize the fear and shame surrounding gray area drinking.

I was proud of myself after sharing my alcohol-free journey, yet I was still wobbly . . . like a young fawn trying to gather her lanky legs into a stride. Getting authentic, real, and vulnerable was a new way for me to find my voice and to lean into who I was becoming. Each conversation about my alcohol-free journey allowed my new skin to begin to grow thicker and stronger. Each day brings a new opportunity to choose again. There is no question which choice is the better one, the one that serves us to become the best versions of ourselves. The other choice, the choice to drink, only steals our joy and robs of us of our time, peace, and clarity.

Finding Your Fun Self Again

By choosing to explore our relationship with alcohol and choosing to be alcohol-free, we communicate to those around us that there is another way to have fun. Many of us have convinced ourselves that the only way we can have fun is by drinking. This just is not true. When you were younger, you had fun when you were not drinking. She is still there within you. You can still be goofy, let loose, and even be the life of the party. The best part is you will remember it all clearly.

One such time was over the summer during the pandemic. My family had been holed up all year, keeping a safe distance from everyone. I decided it would be fun to do something outside that the whole family could enjoy. We ventured out to a water park during the off-hours to avoid the crowds. We climbed inside our inflatable water tubes and relaxed while we drifted around the lazy pool. As we twisted and turned around the pool, the smiles on my children's faces lit up my heart with joy. As we came around the bend, the big waterfalls were dumping water onto those brave enough to go under them. My kids pushed me toward the waterfalls, and for the first time, I didn't worry about what my hair would look like or how freezing cold the water may be as it pummeled down on my head—I just wanted us to have fun. They howled in excitement as their got mom drenched. It was pure fun. Pure joy, where I was clear-minded and present to enjoy every moment of it.

Finding your fun self includes finding healthy ways to come alive. Time near water, especially at the beach, renews my soul. Kayaking allows me to slow down from the fast-paced world and move at the pace of nature. Going back to your childhood memories where you felt joy is key to coming alive again as an adult.

Think back to when you were a little girl. What types of play brought you joy? I always loved riding my bike as a little girl. My pigtails would go flying in the air while pure joy and glee would exude from me as I flew down the streets in my neighborhood. As an adult, riding my road bike brought back that same inner joy. The little girl who felt free and blissful was starting to reappear now.

Instead of punishing myself with a workout for drinking the night before, I was now enjoying my workouts, especially my outdoor bike rides. I created a playlist, called "I Love Me," filled with positive, strong female artists singing songs about our empowerment as women. Now you can find me on bike trails loudly singing these songs as I blaze through trails where my soul comes alive.

Recently, I took a watercolor painting class. I had not painted since I was a young girl. As I sat down and began to paint, I was so immersed in each paint stroke that the to-do list, the worries of life, and the chaos of my day just melted away into the beautiful colors on the paper. I looked up at the clock. Two hours had flown by as I was immersed in pure blissful joy, allowing not only joy but also more expansiveness to enter my soul. This is when you know you are finding your true joy: time disappears, and your little girl comes alive again.

Finding your fun self doesn't mean you *always* need to be doing something. Joy can also be found in rest. During my journey, I started listening to what my body needed, what my spirit craved, and how to reconnect with myself. This took shape in the form of meditation, journaling, hot baths, and long walks with a good podcast—things that allowed my body to rest and unwind like never before. Before then, I did not realize there are seven types of rest, all of which are vital to filling up our buckets.

Here are the seven types of rest, from Saundra Dalton-Smith in her TED Ideas article, "The 7 Types of Rest That Every Person Needs":

- Physical Rest: More sleep, deep breaths, relaxation, and stretching
- Emotional Rest: The space and time to freely express your feelings and cut back on people pleasing—perhaps through journaling and/or therapy
- Mental Rest: Music, meditation, and silence
- Social Rest: Catching up with an old friend or, conversely, taking a break from socializing
- Creative Rest: Reading a book, taking a nature walk
- Spiritual Rest: Doing things that give you sense of purpose or meaning
- Sensory Rest: Turning off devices and screens, finding the quiet[6]

When you're not spending all your time thinking about the next drink, you have more time for life or just to rest. You'll show up in your hobbies, work, parenting, or even rest with more joy, energy, and zest for life. If you are having a hard time figuring out what brings you joy, make a "*not* to-do" list. As you make this *not* to-do list, put everything on it that isn't serving you. You may need to get things out of your life that aren't serving you to make space for the ones that are.

Finally, a great thing to do with your kids or by yourself is a "SWLTY Day." This stands for a "See Where Life Takes You Day," an idea my life coach Cari Rose shared with me as we were tapping back into my joy. A day where you have no plans, no schedule, and let life take you where it wants to.[7]

I recently did a SWLTY Day with my son. We jumped in the car to explore some small little towns nearby. One of them had an airport with a museum. I wasn't even sure if they were open, but we were pleasantly surprised to learn not only were they open but also had a guided tour of two hangers of planes for us to see, a museum, and two outdoor planes to explore. My son was on cloud nine as he *loves* airplanes.

Afterward, we decided to go grab some lunch. We got a little lost but didn't care as we had nowhere to be. We ended up in another adorable little town where we discovered the *best* pizza place. We walked around the town exploring all it had to offer. We let the day take us wherever it wanted. It was one of the most memorable, fun days we have ever had together.

Another way to create simple joy every day is something I call "Find the Beauty in the Day." It can be a simple flower, a sunset, a butterfly . . . something that is beautiful to you. My iPhone camera is full of Find the Beauty in the Day photos. It's a simple way to bring joy and an attitude of gratitude into your day!

It is important to create this joy as you untangle the hard parts of your past. Learning to have fun again without alcohol is possible. Remember, the fun little girl *is* there. She is just waiting for you to dust her off for a good time.

Lie: "Being Sober is Boring."

Truth: Boring is being checked out to all that life has to offer to us. Alcohol does not make us more fun. We had fun when we were younger without any alcohol. When we remove alcohol, it can feel very awkward at first. It takes time and is a process of undoing years of coping mechanisms, trauma responses, and cultural messages. Over time, we see that being alcohol-free allows us to be fully present, joyful, and the truest version of ourselves, not a façade of who we think we are with alcohol. Going back to what made our soul come alive as a child helps us reconnect with ourselves and where we can find joy in our current lives. By finding time for rest and creating joy into our lives, we find our fun selves once again.

Did You Know?

We all want to prevent cancer, yet very few of us discuss or adhere to the warning that alcohol is a known carcinogen. Did you know that alcohol is linked to eight types of cancer? Even though the American Cancer Society recommends not drinking alcohol because there is strong scientific consensus that it causes several types of cancer, as a society we turn our heads the other way. In fact, the evidence indicates that the more alcohol a person drinks—particularly the more alcohol a person drinks regularly over time—the higher his or her risk of developing an alcohol-associated cancer.[8]

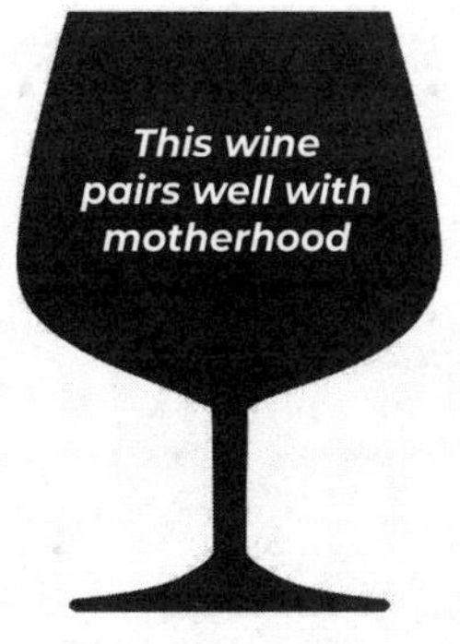

CHAPTER FIVE

"BEHIND EVERY GREAT MOM IS A BOTTLE OF WINE"

I, like so many women, fell deep into the abyss of the intoxicating lies the alcohol industry targeted and marketed to me while I was drinking. I bought the napkins, the T-shirts, the tea towels, even the cups that said things that reinforced my beliefs that alcohol was "Mommy's sanity juice." I could have been the poster child for the mommy wine culture. A year before my exploration on being alcohol-free, I posted a picture on social media of a full glass of wine with a message that read on the glass, "If I go missing, please put my face on wine bottles so my friends know"; the caption sadly proclaimed, "Friday Vibes."

I was literally sucking down the Kool-Aid of pro-drinking messages. I couldn't see that the normative drinking-culture messages were further enforcing that my gray area of drinking was so-called "normal."

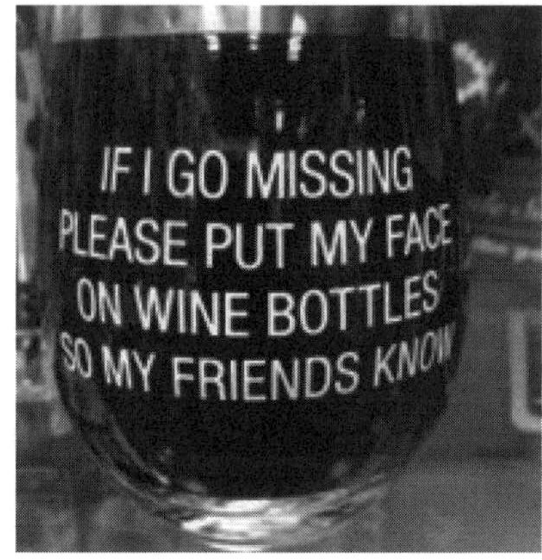

The big alcohol industry—a vast network of producers, distributors, marketers, and retailers—is specifically targeting women with these messages, knowing it is keeping us small, quiet, and checked out. It is particularly disparaging toward moms. We are taught by society that we earned it; we *deserve* it. It is like a mom code we have all gulped down unknowingly.

We trade in playing with our children for the much-deserved beverage society tells us to guzzle to deal with motherhood and all its stresses. We wake up groggy and tired, not giving our best selves to our children or partners. Our fuses are shorter, our anxiety heightened, our depression deepened—all due to alcohol.

But there is no handbook for moms that warns against these side effects of alcohol . . . in fact, it is just the opposite. We are told we will be better moms, better homeschoolers during the pandemic, and better partners stuck in a house together twenty-four seven if we drink.

Even though the alcohol industry and society were telling me drinking was the way to deal with stress, it was definitely not working. They also said drinking, portrayed as a social lubricant of sorts, is the way you connect and celebrate! But the connection was always lost in the blur of a night. I was ashamed that I wanted to come home after Halloween and drink more alone. I was buried in shame that I might have an issue with alcohol. I felt guilty for not being the mother the tea towel said I would be. I felt like a failure because I could not get it under control. Still, I fell for it hook, line, and sinker. I believed it all, like a sheep following its herd. I too had fallen prey to the old, conditioned belief, and there is no shame or guilt in that. Unfortunately, many of us have.

It's been said that with great suffering, there is always great profit. In 2020, total alcoholic beverage sales numbers in the United States reached over $222 billion.[1] The big alcohol industry got moms addicted to the notion that this is how you deal with motherhood's challenges. My lens was so fogged, so unclear (with no clear path ahead), that even I could not see that my joy, happiness, and time with my family was being plundered by alcohol. All I could see was gray, but it was the only color I knew on a day in, day out basis, so it seemed normal.

As I awoke to this manipulation in my alcohol-free journey, I realized for the first time that I had become slowly imprisoned over time by the subtle falsehoods that had taken root into my psyche. My shame and guilt started to melt away as anger filled their place. I am angry at the alcohol industry for serving us a known carcinogenic without a warning label. I am angry that we are not taught this information until we search it out. They have planted a vast garden of pitcher plants knowing the dangers, leaving it up to *us* to navigate our way out of this hellish garden.

The worst part is we are helping the alcohol industry unintentionally by pushing the pitcher plant upon each other in so many obscure, insidious ways. When we post a picture of a drink on social media, we are putting alcohol on a pedestal; when we put together a so-called "care package" or a basket filled with alcohol, insinuating, *This will take care of you*; or when we buy the mommy wine-culture napkins, cups, and T-shirts as gifts for our friends, we are implying to other moms that this is how you deal with motherhood. When we buy, wear, decorate, and post these normative pro-drinking messages (such as "My Kids Whine, So I Wine"), we are not only perpetuating the problem for other women but also actually *endorsing* the big alcohol industry. (Remember that the best form of advertising is word of mouth . . . a recommendation from a trusted friend!)

Once I started waking up to all of these subliminal pro-drinking messages around me, I could not unsee them. They are everywhere, and they are making us sick. I gathered up all of my pro-drinking knickknacks and threw them in the trash—where they belonged!

No, I am not here to shame us. We are conditioned to believe this lie—that behind every great mom is a bottle of wine. We can have compassion for ourselves in that we were using alcohol thinking it would solve a problem for us, but we *know* better.

One day at lunch, I sat outside at a restaurant on a beautiful, sunny day. The warm breeze blew through my hair as I ate my salad. A mother and her teenage daughter walked up, sitting near me to enjoy a mother-daughter luncheon. The mother had a T-shirt on that said in all caps, "ALL YOU NEED IS WINE."

I sat there staring at the mother, not with judgment but with empathy as she, too, had fallen prey to the marketing trap. I wanted to go up to her table and hug her and tell her I used to believe the same thing, but that I learned the hard way that it isn't *true*! But what struck me the most was that I could not stop wondering what her teenage daughter was thinking. Her biggest female role model in her life, her mother, was subliminally telling her: *All you really need, sweetie, is wine to deal with it all.* It broke my heart for both of them Do we really want to tell our children to deal with life's challenges with alcohol? What our children need is a mother who knows how to truly care for herself and can regulate her nervous system.

Another cultural assumption is that we *all* drink. This became more apparent to me at work during the first months of the COVID-19 pandemic at a national sales meeting, one held virtually due to the lockdown.

The day of our sales meeting, a box from my company arrived at my door. Excitedly, I opened the box and found a small bottle of champagne, with a note that said "To toast the winners" while listening online to who won the sales awards. In the past, I would have cracked that puppy open and enjoyed it during the call, not giving it a second thought. Now I was looking at it, perplexed. If I were someone in recovery who could not have alcohol in their house, it had just been automatically delivered to my door—with no questions asked. It's just a presumption—a given—that we all drink.

I threw it in the trash can, knowing I did not need it to celebrate after being alcohol-free for many months at that point. I wondered, though, about those who may not have been able to throw it away. Was that unexpected gift nothing more than an invitation to begin drinking again?

I do not care if someone chooses to drink: that is their choice. Nor am I trying to exude any moral superiority. My goal is simply to start a conversation on why we normalize drinking as much as we stigmatize it! This juxtaposition creates *so* much shame around our drinking. We blame and punish ourselves for choosing what everyone has told us is "normal" drinking. It's all so confusing that we struggle silently—unsure of ourselves.

A "Quarantini" Is Essential

I had been embarking on this sober-curious journey for several months with questions, fear, and uncertainty when the world came to a complete halt in March 2020. I was grateful to be past the physical detox phase when the pandemic hit. As I was learning how to feel my feelings for the first time, I knew the anxiety from the pandemic coupled with alcohol would have only propelled me even further down that "one-way drinking highway."[2] At the same time, the seemingly nonstop COVID-19 coverage on TV, radio, and social media reared its ugly head, only exacerbating our fears as we were trapped inside our homes. There was no running off to work or going shopping to distract from what was happening with the virus. The world had come to a screeching halt.

And when everything stopped, we were all left staring straight into the face of our feelings.

Some of us could not handle it and chose addictive substances to check out and not deal with it all, while others looked head-on into those feelings of fear and uncertainty. I had already chosen the latter path a few months back and now was faced with navigating this alcohol-free path with the world's fears coupled with my own.

Memes on social media were encouraging those who did not know how to handle the uncertainty and fear of the pandemic to just wash it all down with a "Quarantini." Society, which normalizes this highly addictive drug, was now showing up on social media claiming that day drinking was more normal than ever. You cannot go to work; you are stuck all day inside with your children and your spouse—nowhere to go, nowhere to run—so society told us once again to drink to escape it all.

With the lockdown in place and only essential businesses open, it was not ironic at all that our society deemed liquor stores as "essential businesses." *Let the addiction grow—it's essential, like our groceries and mail, right?* For the first time, you could get a margarita to go from a restaurant. Did individuals really wait until they got home to drink it? I am guessing most drank it on their way home with their takeout—not only dangerous in terms of feeding the addiction but also for our safety on the roads.

"Alcohol will relax you" was the subtle, unsaid fabrication carefully embedded into commercials and social media posts, especially during the pandemic. It is easy to grab a drink and just want to check out to it all. But the reality was this message was driving up our addiction rates in our country at an alarming rate. Alcohol sales went up by 32 percent during the pandemic.[3]

For women, it is even worse, according to the National Institute of Alcohol Abuse and Alcoholism:

> For people experiencing stress from unemployment to feelings of isolation during physical distancing, the COVID-19 emergency may be influencing alcohol consumption for many reasons. In several studies, increases in drinking were more likely for women, particularly those reporting increases in stress. Women have been affected more, in a variety of ways, by the pandemic due to increased responsibilities as they care for children and families—often while still working—in addition to the loss of more jobs and income than men, and preexisting differences in pay and in the number of single-parent homes led by women. These stressors are associated with more alcohol use among women.[4]

"There's been a 41 percent increase in heavy drinking days among women since the onset of the pandemic," adds the *Journal of the American Medical Association*.[5]

I heard from so many of my friends who said, "I drank so much more during the pandemic, and it scared me." Not surprising since we were carrying so much weight all while trying to find balance in our lives. Coupled with the madness of suddenly being a homeschooler and trying to balance work all at the same time, these messages of "You will be a better mom if you drink" were shown repeatedly on television shows, commercials, and social media. Like the meme that showed a mom with a shopping cart full of back-to-school supplies that included pens, pencils, paper, and a case of wine, telling us in essence that you'll be a better homeschooler with tons of wine (and, by the way, will be hungover for your children's morning Zoom classes). I cannot think of anything worse. Trying to juggle my work, my kids' classes, making nonstop meals in the kitchen, and cleaning—all while being in a fogged hangover—would have been like adding fuel to the fire during the pandemic.

WebMD reported, "We found the largest increase occurred in women with children under the age of five, who were at home. This population doubled or tripled drinking quantities."[6]

There were so many reasons to drink now that the world was in chaos. The fear of job loss, homeschooling, health, and the deep political divide would have only increased my few glasses a night. Thinking that alcohol was a warm blanket providing comfort during these challenges would have been another myth that I would have fallen into by conforming to society.

But, like a gift, the pandemic was also an easier time to become alcohol-free because there weren't any parties to go to, no celebrations or get-togethers. The temptation was eliminated by the lockdown. Being stuck inside allowed me the time and space to surf the crave with a good nonalcoholic beer or a good book.

The pandemic was a mixed bag, bringing out the worst in some of us and the best in others. Days turned into months of waiting to know when it was safe to venture out, where we could go, and whom we could see. For an instant gratification society, this was a huge challenge to just wait. To sit and wait with patience before venturing into an unknown environment of who knows what. Humans are creatures of connection, routine, and certainty—none of which were available to any of us. We were left with the choice to navigate this unfamiliar landscape equipped with either the facts and truth or fear and uncertainty. Our normal was gone, and no one even knew how or when normal would reappear.

I could see now on the flipside of alcohol that these falsehoods, memes, and even the normalization of day drinking during the quarantine were not going to serve our society well. It would be so easy (like the Staples Easy Button) to reach for a drink to numb out the fear of not enough toilet paper, fear of supply chain issues, or just a fear of death itself from COVID-19. Our selfish hoarding instincts took over, many of us fearing that there just would not be enough for all of us. We were glued to our TV and phones for what was to come next, but we were only left with more fear and uncertainty about the future. While waiting for answers, many of us fell further into addiction, believing that the solution would emerge from the bottom of the bottle.

Since choosing to be alcohol-free, I spent my days in the quarantine outside in nature, where taking long walks listening to podcasts became my daily therapy. One of my favorite podcasts during this time was American professor, lecturer, author, and podcast host Brené Brown's *Unlocking Us*, where she discussed "Anxiety, Calm, and Over-/Under-Functioning."

As I was unlocking parts of myself that had been hidden away and masked by doing and not feeling, her truth on anxiety set me free. I realized I had been using alcohol as one more distraction to deal with my anxiety. Almost every woman in my sobriety group described themselves as a "high-functioning person": someone who usually runs on high anxiety or who, when in crisis, goes into caretaking mode—*doing*—thereby controlling the situation. Those who are "under functioning" leave it to someone else to take charge.

Brené, who is also sober, unlocks the truth on how high functioning puts us into a "doing mode" versus a "feeling mode."[7] I could now see that even though I had been alcohol-free for some time, it could be easy to replace alcohol with distractions of doing, rescuing, and trying to control situations . . . just like I had in the past. Moms are constantly on the go; distractions are a part of our very fiber whether we like or not.

In some cosmic way, the quarantine and the ability to work from home allowed more space and time to open up for this journey of self-discovery. The inner work takes a lot of time, but now the Universe had made that available to me. I did not take it for granted that I had time to pause and reflect on my feelings and choices. It forced all of us to slow down. Slowing down and not being distracted by a thousand things to do was exactly what my soul needed at that point. In fact, during this time, I spent many hours in state parks because it was the only place you could go safely throughout the lockdown.

The greatest awakening during the pandemic for me was that our health is our wealth. One of my main whys for staying alcohol-free was to be the healthiest and best version of myself. I knew that every morning I woke up deflated, at a deficit from the wine the night before, that started my immune system, brain, and body at a deficit as well. I could feel my mind, body, and spirit shifting into alignment for the first time in my life.

Connection with my Sober Sis group was also key because the pandemic made it very easy to isolate. As the British-Swiss writer and journalist Johann Hari says in his TED talk, "The antidote to addiction is connection."[8]

I was so grateful the ten of us had access to a network of women from all over the world that was available twenty-four seven and also a smaller, more intimate group on Marco Polo. This was vital to forging forward in our alcohol-free lifestyle. True self-care is not manicures, facials, and flowers but a community of likeminded women who at any given moment were there for each other. A safe place where we could be seen, heard, and held—that is *true* self-care.

Making It Public

As I approached one year alcohol-free, I was starting to settle into less doing and more just *being*. My thick, new skin had grown over the past 365 days alcohol-free into a flexible, strong shield . . . and it was time to be seen. I knew I needed to shift out of my little bubble of only close friends and family who knew I was alcohol-free. It was time to put it out there on social media. I knew I needed to do this to keep myself accountable. I also wanted to help other women who were stuck in the gray area of the "detox just to retox" loop.[9] My anxiety washed over me with thoughts of *What will people say if I mess up down the road? What if, what if, what if?*

As Brené Brown says,

> If you are not in the arena getting your ass kicked on occasion, I am not interested in or open to your feedback. There are a million cheap seats in the world today filled with people who will never be brave with their own lives but will spend every ounce of energy they have hurling advice and judgment at those of us trying to dare greatly. Their only contributions are criticism, cynicism, and fearmongering. If you're criticizing from a place where you're not also putting yourself on the line, I'm not interested in your feedback.[10]

I knew it was time to step into the arena. It was time to speak up and go against the grain and the masses.

It was time, as Brené Brown says, to "dare greatly."

So one year after this alcohol-free journey began, I posted on Instagram:

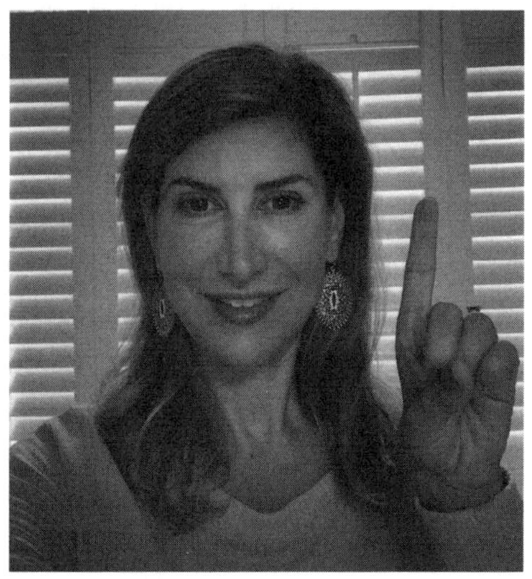

> One year ago today, I had my last drink. A little over a year ago, I started questioning my relationship with alcohol. I never drank during the day or hit a rock bottom, but rather felt trapped in the "detox just to retox" loop.[11] I can drink anytime I want to, but now I choose not to after learning what alcohol was doing to my mind, body, and spirit over this past year. I am more clear-minded in all aspects of my life, more present with my loved ones, have more energy, and a greater sense of who I am and why I am worth it. I don't post this for kudos but rather for anyone else who is questioning it and wants to be free from the mental mind game of gray area drinking.

As I hit share, I rolled out my mat to do yoga. I didn't want to check my phone every few minutes like my recovering, inner people pleaser was telling me to do so. After my yoga session, I picked up my phone to see tons of support from my friends. I knew if I kept this to myself and did not share it, I was only perpetuating the stigma associated with it. I wished someone had posted something like this in my circle while a war was raging within my head, when I was thinking I was alone and crazy.

Part of me couldn't believe I had made it to one year. It had been a beautiful year of discovering so much about of myself, yet this small jokester-like voice still existed in my head. Even though I had not one sip of alcohol, the jokester was still lurking around in the dark spaces in my mind with the question of *Could I ever go back to just drinking on occasion*? I knew the truth, I knew the dangers, yet my mind would wonder off to a place where deprivation still lurked.

At a year, these thoughts were far and few between as the days progressed, but they popped up from time to time . . . that was, until it all came crashing down.

The Lie: "Behind Every Great Mom Is a Bottle of Wine"

The Truth*:* Behind every great mom is a true sense of who she is. It is not your fault you have fallen into the alcohol trap, but it is your responsibility to navigate your way out. We have been conditioned by a societal and cultural belief that all our challenges, uncertainty, and fears can be solved by using alcohol as a crutch. We have been hooked into believing the intoxicating lies of alcohol will make us better mothers, partners, and professionals. Once we can see the truth, we cannot unsee it.

Did You Know?

"The sober movement is growing. Several reports forecast that the global market for nonalcoholic drinks will grow by 32 percent to $30 billion by 2025. The more non-alcoholic options we provide and give as an alternative as a society, the more we reinforce that being alcohol-free is a normal choice. Long gone are the days of only one non-alcoholic beer as an option, now you can find alcohol-free tequilas, gins, and even wines."

—Richie Crowley (@rickieticklez)[12]

CHAPTER SIX

"GO AHEAD, YOU CAN HAVE A SIP"

Even though Stacy had told me moderation did not work for her at the beginning of our reset, she had now convinced herself during her second 21-Day Reset, after a year of not drinking, that she could just have sips. She said that she didn't really like it but that a sip would not hurt anything. I was perplexed, to say the least. I kept asking her, "If you don't like it or need it, then why take a sip?"

She felt that after healing her inner work, she could now be a take-it-or-leave-it drinker after not drinking for more than a year. We all looked at her in amazement. She had achieved what we all thought we had longed for: a take-it-or-leave-it relationship with alcohol. I wondered: *Can you be cured of this tricky gray area drinking like she had? Was it possible after a year and half of not drinking?*

My inner knowing was yelling back to my brain, *No way*, but the jokester was peering out, asking, *Well, maybe*?

Over the next few months, I found myself second-guessing my inner knowing once again. I trusted Stacy: She was my go-to person within our online SoberMinded Sisterhood. Stacy and I had relied heavily on each other throughout our alcohol-free journey. So when she announced after a year of not drinking that she could take it or leave it with sips, my brain immediately started to perk up with *Can we do this too? Maybe we* are *cured—it's been a year and half*!

Even with all the education on the science of alcohol, all the transformative shifts that had occurred, at times all these shifts related to being alcohol-free can be overwhelming. Meanwhile, life's big challenges don't stop.

One such night, the kids were torturing our anxious little dog, Phoebe. I repeatedly asked them to stop, but after being trapped in our house for almost a year with the pandemic, Phoebe became their outlet for play. This increased Phoebe's anxiety and would make her cling to me even more. After many more requests for them to stop agonizing her, I lost it and yelled at them both to give me their phones and go to their rooms.

As I looked at my eleven-year-old son's phone, I found nothing of interest, so I put in on my dresser. As I opened my fourteen-year-old daughter's phone, I saw a Snapchat with her best friend where they were discussing how they tried "nic," which, unbeknownst to me at the time, is vaping. I was floored when I learned what it was. Ashley is a track and cross-country runner, and she is vaping?! Then her best friend went on about trying "alc"—alcohol.

I asked Ashley to come into my room to discuss this Snapchat conversation between her and her best friend. Ashley told me her cousin gave her the vaping pen and she had only taken a few puffs.

She promised me she had not tried drinking. We had a long conversation about the dangers and addictions of both vaping and alcohol. I called my sister afterward to let her know her son, Ashley's cousin, had introduced her to vaping.

My sister replied, "I hate to tell you this, but it is not true. We got a different story. Ashley brought her own vaping pen."

I was floored once again. I know at this age they are going to try things, but the lying I could not handle. I asked Ashley to come back into my room, this time asking her to tell me the truth. She said she was scared to tell me that she bought the vaping pen from a boy up the street for twenty dollars. I felt like a complete failure as a mother. Had I not taught her to not buy things from strangers?! I told her that the boy could have put anything into the vaping pen and either gotten her very sick or, worse yet, killed her.

But I was most upset about the lying.

A few days after this incident, I began to feel overwhelmed by everything. It all felt like too much. Fighting for over a year to stay alcohol-free. Fighting about politics with my husband. Fighting with my kids over COVID-19 rules to keep us safe. Fighting to turn around the sales in my new territory, which was now virtual.

It was like I was at war with everyone around me, but now I was beginning to doubt my own self again. I started to question the way I was showing up to everyone in my COVID-19 bubble. It felt like no one seemed to like me for the past year, and now I was beginning to wonder what all the fight was for.

I sank into a deep, dark place in my mind. Tears of anguish washed over me. I didn't see the point of fighting anymore. I walked down to our basement, grabbed a bottle of red wine, and poured a big glass for myself.

The first drink in fifteen months.

I took a big swig. It burned going down, and my stomach perked right up shouting, *What the hell are we doing*? It did not feel good at all. My stomach churned, but I was in so much emotional pain that I just didn't want to feel it anymore. I didn't want to decide on the discipline for the kids, I didn't want to try to explain my political views, I didn't want to decide what was for dinner anymore, I didn't want to hear that I lost another case at work and there was nothing I could do. I didn't want to decide who could go where safely within our COVID-19 protocols. I just wanted to escape it all, hit the Easy Button, and check out.

I was having my first "F*ck-It Moment."

I had taken three sips of my glass of merlot when Paul came down to the basement to ask what I was doing. He gently said, "I didn't realize how much pain you were in; you don't have to drink."

But I was numb to him. And I just wanted to continue numbing. I didn't want to feel any of it anymore.

I stared at the big glass of red wine and said, "I think I will just go back to the way I used to be—checked out. Everyone liked me more that way. I didn't catch the kids misbehaving; I didn't get into arguments with you because I really didn't care about what was going on in the world. I functioned okay at work. No one felt like they were *in trouble* with me back then, so why not just go back?"

Just as I finished saying all that to Paul, Ashley came around the corner and saw the big glass of red wine in front of me on the table. With tears in her eyes, she asked, "Is this my fault?"

It was like my why slapped me across my face. Here I am making an unhealthy choice. A choice that will have consequences. How can I drink this glass of wine when I am telling her it's gasoline, a drug that's highly addictive? How can I preach to her to not vape, to avoid addictive substances, yet here I am modeling just the opposite?

In that moment, I realized I had to choose my why again—to be the best version of myself. To be a present mother. I got up and poured the glass of wine down the drain in the sink. I sat back down with Ashley and said, "I had a choice. Initially, I made the wrong choice, but then I made a better choice. I am human and I am not perfect. But we all get another chance to make the right choice. To forgive our mistakes and learn from them." We hugged each other, knowing we both learned that we needed to be honest with ourselves, our feelings, and our choices.

The next night, I was astonished to find the exact taste of the merlot I had sipped yesterday was in my mouth again at the 5 p.m. wine hour. Even though it had been over a year of not one sip of alcohol, my brain and body were back and ready for their regular 5 p.m. dopamine hit. This wine taste in my mouth from just three sips of alcohol the day before made me realize how addictive this stuff really is. This sidestep taught me that even "sips" were an insidiously easy way back down into the pitcher plant. I had not trusted my inner knowing, got caught up in the trickiness of believing I too was cured from gray area drinking, and able to handle sips.

Shortly after my sip incident, Stacy came back on Marco Polo announcing that her sips of alcohol over time had led her back down a mental mind game with alcohol that she had prayed her way out of. She explained to our group that her sip-sidesteps had led her back to thinking about drinking almost nightly. Alcohol even in small amounts plays a big role on the effects of our brain. Stacy described to us on Marco Polo this perfect analogy of how believing she could take sips of alcohol or moderate her drinking played tricks with her mind:

> The lies alcohol tells me so easily make me forget the truths. Alcohol is like an abusive ex-boyfriend. You know he is no good for you anymore and so you do the hard work to break up with him. You tell yourself *I am worth more, I deserve better.* You tell yourself *I am better without him.* I can get healthy and do all the work, but it doesn't change my abusive boyfriend. When he comes back around with his charming ways, he says to you this time will be different. He is the funniest, most charismatic guy in the room. He makes you start to think he is different now and maybe we can be together again. You think to yourself, *I am different now too, so maybe this time it will be different,* but the reality is he is still the same guy. Slowly, over time, his old ways and abusive patterns reappear.
>
> This is what it is like with alcohol. You want to believe it will be different this time. That this time you will be in control of alcohol, you can have a healthy relationship with alcohol, but it is not the case.

These sidesteps, or, as we call them in Sober Sis, "data points," were moving us further down the alcohol-free exit ramp on the "one-way drinking highway."[1] As Jenn Kautsch says, "Data points are just valuable feedback, not a setback."[2] Each data point was preparing us, training us and our minds to choose to remain alcohol-free. Even though we each had evolved into healthier versions of ourselves, alcohol was still the same old bad ex-boyfriend. Telling ourselves that we had changed, evolved, or transformed did not mean that our brains, minds, or spirits would no longer fall prey to alcohol's abusive ways. Thankfully, I did not go back to "Day One" in my alcohol-free journey after this incident. It was just another day moving me forward in my alcohol-free continuum.

Author William Porter of *Alcohol Explained* describes why even after years of abstaining from alcohol, our minds and mental triggers don't forget:

> As the mental triggers still remain, no matter how long someone has stopped for, it is only a matter of time before they end up right where they were when they stopped drinking. Their mind has learnt, many years before, through constant repetition, that another drink will alleviate that unpleasant feeling. It has learnt that and it will never be forgotten . . . their mind will remember the lesson, and even after twenty, thirty, or even forty years, it will still remember, and if they have a drink ever again their mind will set in motion a craving for alcohol."[3]

After this sidestep, I came to the realization that I no longer wanted this substance to be dangling in front of me as something that maybe one day I'd be able to moderate. A shift into finally trusting my inner knowing. I had doubted my inner knowing when I took those few sips. I questioned my own intuition and reentered the mental mind game with myself once again. Seeing Stacy come back around from her own sidestep allowed me to reflect on the importance of trusting myself even when others I looked up to on the same journey took their sidesteps.

As Glennon Doyle tells us in her *Get Untamed: The Journal (How to Quit Pleasing and Start Living)*,

> Our deep desires are wise, true, beautiful, and things we can grant ourselves without abandoning our Knowing. Following our deep desire always returns us to integrity. If your desire feels wrong to you: Go deeper. You can trust yourself. You just have to get low enough. So, a nightly desire for a bottle of wine? If your Knowing doesn't trust it,

> it's just a surface desire. A surface desire is one that conflicts with our Knowing. We must ask our surface desires: What is the desire beneath this desire? Is it rest? Is it peace?[4]

At the surface lies perfection, not enough-ism, and over functioning, keeping the external show going, but deep down there is a woman who is not divided and who knows what she needs.

I woke up the next day after being in the same pajamas for two days with a new perspective. Each day we get to make a choice, the right choice for ourselves. The easy choice is to check out, which solves nothing and adds fuel to the fire. It's a choice to get up and fight for yourself once again. I realized after talking to my sister and my therapist that not everyone is going to like the new you or the way you show up, but being true to you and living authentically is the most important choice. Not everyone will like it, but their reaction is not for me.

We also need to remind ourselves that when we have sidesteps in our alcohol-free journey, our culture tells us we are failures, that we are not enough. But they are there to teach us, to give us feedback and guidance, moving us forward on our own unique journey.

During this unraveling of my perfectionism, I started allowing myself to show up "messier" and more authentic, foregoing the role of "I have to control this." I no longer want to control everything or look like everything's perfect. I was beginning to embark on the most beautiful part of the journey, yielding in more serenity, less drama, more rest, and less doing. It was a relief to let go.

Facing Our Pasts

Now that alcohol was gone for some time, the traumas each of us in our Sober Sis group had experienced in life started to resurface like oil in water. It was becoming clear that each of us had a painful story of suffering that needed to be healed. Each of us was leaning on alcohol to ease the burden, erase the pain, and to check out of reality.

Each day we would make a video on Marco Polo, responding to the other women's vulnerable videos with support, validation, alignment, and encouragement. Each of us could see ourselves in one another. The shame, guilt, and regret started to dissipate as we could see each of us was trying to cope with life's challenges.

Elizabeth describes how her drinking transitioned from a social to a nightly escape because she felt like she needed it:

> About eight years ago, life got very difficult for me. I had a lot of stress in my life already because I have a large family with seven children, and just being a mom is stressful enough, but then my husband almost died. It was my husband, Tim's, fiftieth birthday and I was setting up a surprise birthday party for him while my boys took him go-karting. I had invited over a hundred people to our house, something I had never done before. I got a phone call while setting up for the party that Tim had had an aortic aneurysm. He was rushed to the hospital, where they gave him a 1 percent chance of surviving. His aorta aneurysm was caused by an aortic dissection. Tim was in a coma for two weeks. During this same time, one of my sons was diagnosed with bipolar disorder. Thankfully, Tim pulled through, but my son attempted suicide twice. Plus, our adopted children were also experiencing some trauma-related issues from their past. It was all too much all at once. After taking care of everyone all day, I would sit down with my rewarding glass of wine. I felt like it was the

> only way to get through it all. I looked forward to it at the end of each day, which became a nightly habit for me over time. Over time, I realized I was always looking forward to a drink anywhere I went and then realized this was not okay. It was my crutch and my reward.

To this day, Elizabeth has remained alcohol-free in our journey together, but many of the women in my group continued to struggle in their efforts to stay alcohol-free. Each Marco Polo post on someone's sidestep was like wind in our sails, pushing us further along in our alcohol-free journey, learning from one another.

Lisa from our group describes her struggle to remain alcohol-free:

> Even after doing the 21-Day Reset, followed by a 90-day alcohol-free program, then an intensive (read, expensive) small-group coaching initiative, I continued to drink on and off. It was the person Veronica Valli of *Soberful Life* spoke of pertaining to people with drinking problems. You are always doing one of three things: drinking, thinking about drinking, or thinking about not drinking.[5] I'd wake up with a hangover and then think about not drinking, chastising and shaming myself for most of the day. I had done it again—failed. Then, as the Tylenol did its job and things didn't seem so bleak, I thought about drinking. I put aside my hangover, ignored what I had promised myself—and others—and thought about how and when I would drink that evening. Then I drank. That was my daily cycle, the rhythm of my life.

We all chimed in on Marco Polo, reassuring Lisa she was not a failure. These sidesteps in the group were like a game of whack-a-mole, where the perfection monster would pop his ugly head out with his swords of shame and guilt, but collectively we would whack him back into his place, reminding whoever had a sidestep that she was not a failure, but that rather it was a data point on her journey. Like the old saying goes, "Progress over perfection." Each time one of us would be lured back to the intoxicating lies alcohol whispered to our brain, we would learn from that woman's post on what continuing drinking brought her or, I should say, did *not* bring her. It was all feedback, never a failure.

These sidesteps are like training for a marathon, as author Holly Whitaker describes in her book *Quit Like a Woman*. One would never just get up and run the New York City Marathon. You train for it, building up to each additional mile, each run giving you feedback, pushing you along in your training from running zero to twenty-six miles.

Many of us who decide to go alcohol-free think we have to be perfect with abstaining from alcohol from the get-go. Not so, says Holly Whitaker:

> The last thing you need when you're trying to quit drinking is stress and being told that your success on this path is measured by your (perfect, seamless) abstinence, or that you must go back to square one if you drink while trying to quit, only makes you feel more helpless, more defeated, and therefore more in need of a drink.[6]

Whenever one of the women in my group would drink, they would always say, "I got busy, and I stopped doing the work." Alcohol can be much like the Staples Easy Button: It is an easy way to check out. It is easy to go back to the way things were—but we must also remember: *the old ways weren't working.* We all want instant relief, instant gratification from life's stresses and challenges.

We have been trained by society to seek instant relief and avoid pain. This is the very hook that trapped us—the instant relief we got from alcohol, yet it adds to our pain.

A new shift was blossoming in me to no longer wanting or needing a substance to celebrate or to escape. A shift out of wondering if one day in the future I could be a take-it-or-leave-it drinker. (The irony is that true take-it-or-leave-it drinkers don't ever even think about moderating).

Keeping that thought in my mind was leaving me in a purgatory that was not serving me. I knew moderation of any sort was circling the top of the pitcher plant, where at any moment when life got too hard, I would slide right back down into its sweet nectar. The pull and tug of alcohol lurking around the corner ready to overtake my mind, body, and spirit once again was no longer an option. I knew that moderation was allowing the mental tug of war to reappear, and to keep it at bay would be constant work. In that, there is no freedom. I would be a slave to the guardrails put in place to try to achieve moderation, only to allow the mental tug of war to take over my brain once again.

This shift was so strong and brought me such an inner peace, knowing that I hold the power to connect and celebrate with others. I no longer needed alcohol to escape the pain, which allowed space for inner peace to resonate so strongly because no one and nothing could ever take it away from me. Sure, this means sitting with the icky feelings and not padding myself, but it also means dealing with them versus just numbing them to be dealt with later. More importantly, I had finally shifted away from the deprivation mindset and any notion that I would even want to entertain a substance that provides no benefit and disconnects me from myself. I no longer felt I needed it anymore.

It was becoming clearer for me in this alcohol-free journey that if I took the time to heal the inner suffering parts of myself, then I would no longer need to reach for the wine bottle.

The Lie: "Go Ahead, You Can Have a Sip"

The Truth: Go ahead, trust yourself. You know what's best for you. Even after having time and space between us and alcohol, our minds never forget the illusions we used to believe about alcohol. It is easy to fall back into the pitcher plant's trap of deceit when we never hit rock bottom. It takes hard work, discipline, and debunking the beliefs about ourselves and alcohol to move past it. Once we can see this truth, deprivation goes away because we no longer want to choose a lie, a myth, or an illusion that alcohol provides a crutch or a reward. Sidesteps in our journey provide meaningful feedback pushing us forward on our alcohol-free journey if we learn from them and don't give up.

Did You Know?

"Within eight weeks of remaining alcohol-free, your liver sheds excess fat and resumes normal liver functions."[7]

—Annie Grace

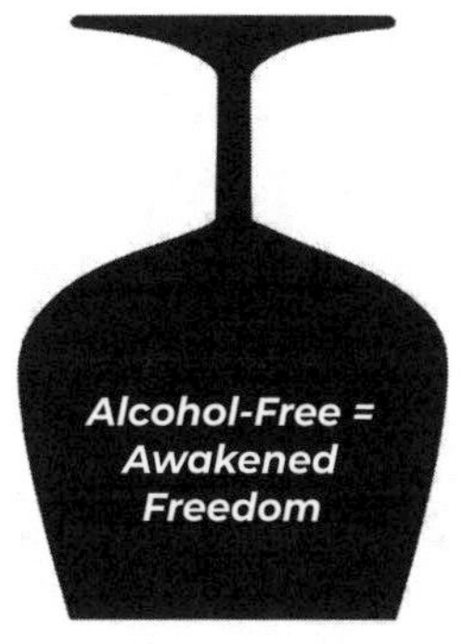

CHAPTER SEVEN

THE END OF THE MERRY-GO-ROUND RIDE

We had not seen my dad in over two years because of COVID-19. But over Thanksgiving 2021, my brother, sister, and I, along with our families, traveled the long six-hour flight and two-hour drive to see my dad and my stepmom in Washington state. I had forgotten that the last time I saw my dad, I was still drinking. Upon our arrival, my dad welcomed me with big open arms, saying, "I got you guys two cases of wine for your Airbnb."

Even though I had told him I had stopped drinking, he had forgotten. I gently reminded him, "I no longer drink, Dad." He replied, "Oh yeah, that's right."

Each of us came with our own expectations of the trip, each expectation different and each not discussed. As we settled into our Airbnb, I was now keenly aware (with no fog distracting my lens) of each of the roles my brother, sister, and I played in our family dynamics.

My brother is the laid-back, spontaneous adventurer who always loved a last-minute idea. My sister, the in-between, take-it-or-leave-it, go-with-the-flow peacemaker was the glue that held our family together. Then there was me, the type A planner and caretaker.

The first day, I noticed everyone kept coming to me, asking me, "What are we going to do today?" In the past, I would have been on autopilot, never giving my role much thought. I would have just fulfilled my part as usual. Now in my second year of sobriety and newfound awareness, I found myself no longer wanting to be the "organizer in chief" or the caregiver for everyone. No longer was I trying to meet everyone's expectations. The feeling of trying to make everyone happy and now realizing it was impossible left me with even more bitterness and resentment. I tried to express that everyone should do what they wanted to do, but my "people" expected me to show up like I always had. My old ways crept back into my autopilot coping mechanisms. I Googled the weather and looked up nearby hiking parks to help everyone have a great day. My wise younger sister (who has always felt like my older sister to me) caught me in all this "doing" and said, "You said you don't want to be the planner, the caretaker, but here you are texting us the weather and where to go."

She was right. I was doing what I always did, taking care of everyone else, putting their needs before my own. Like an invisible map, with known coordinates that I have flown over and over again,

I was showing up in the expected role I had played my entire life with my family and then experiencing resentment afterward.

We have so many invisible roles in our lives, the ones we play in our homes on a daily basis, the ones we show up in for friends, the role we play at work. We rarely even think about these roles, we just play them. The way we show up is expected by our family, friends, and coworkers.

In the past, I would have taken all that resentment and bitterness of my expected caretaker and planner role and drowned it in a big glass of red wine at the end of the day. Alcohol was the place where I washed down the yucky feelings of perfectionism and chronic people pleasing at the end of the day. The truth was so vividly clear to me now: In the past, alcohol had silenced my inner knowing that was desperately trying to say, *I don't want these expectations, they aren't serving me*. I knew if I had chosen a drink to drown it all out, it would have kept me trapped into that role. Silencing what I truly needed and wanted. Keeping the chronic people pleaser in motion.

My old vices still pop up all the time. Healing them looks like letting them go repeatedly. Being aware and *not* letting those old patterns and habits get away with it anymore is the transformation. It's catching them more. It doesn't look perfect. It takes practice. It's reflecting on what I truly want, what brings me joy and, as my wise sister says, stating my preferences or boundaries to voice what I really want.

Yung Pueblo, author of *Clarity & Connection*, gives us the grace we all need to give ourselves: "Next time you feel agitated because you are falling back into your past patterns, remember that simply being aware that you have fallen back into repeating the past is a sign of progress. Self-awareness comes before the great leap forward in your personal transformation."[1]

F*ck-It Moments

While in lockdown, my family and I had planned a trip to Aruba for 2021. It was the light at the end of tunnel after the strict COVID bubble we had created to keep our family safe.

We arrived in Aruba, excited to do all the activities we had booked during lockdown the year before. We went on an UTV tour exploring the island in a metal contraption that scared the shit of out me, but we were all laughing and finally having fun together.

Christmas Day, as I slept in the hotel bed with my daughter, my leg touched hers, and I realized she was burning up. *Shit,* I thought, *she has a raging fever.*

Ashley woke up feeling awful, congested, and just plain miserable. I had brought a few COVID tests with me, so the first thing I did was test her. It was negative. Whew. *Okay, she must have the horrible cold that had just circulated throughout our house,* I thought. The next day, she felt better after spending the entirety of Christmas Day in bed in Aruba. We went on with our excursions for the next few days. Thankfully, everything we did was outside.

All too soon, it was time to test to go home. After our tests, the lab said it would take several hours to get our results and that they would email them to us.

Later that day, I was swimming in the hotel's pool when my husband came to the edge of the pool. He leaned down to me in the pool and said, "You have to see our test results."

My stomach clenched. I jumped out the of pool to look at his phone. The email read "positive" for Ashley.

We immediately grabbed our things and headed back to our hotel room. We called the front desk; they said that since my husband and son were negative, they could fly home the next day to the US . . . and would I be quarantining with my daughter?

With Paul and Grant on their way home, Ashley and I bunkered in our hotel room, playing cards and watching movies.

Quarantining together was a blessing in disguise because our relationship had been severed by COVID when it first broke out. Ashley, the social butterfly, always had me worried sick about getting the family ill with COVID because she wanted to see everyone all the time. This left the two of us butting heads numerous times over the past year and half. Now quarantined in Aruba, we were rekindling and bonding once again.

I knew there was a great chance I could get COVID from her and then we would have to stay another week in Aruba. The uncertainty of the situation was overwhelming, let alone navigating the technicalities of getting out of Aruba if we were both negative.

I needed to know if I had COVID, so I went to the hotel's testing lab to find out. After fifteen minutes, the healthcare provider walked over to me and said, "You are negative." Total relief washed over me. I knew now that if Ashley tested negative tomorrow, we could both fly home since it had been five days since her symptoms began. Per CDC guidelines, that made her travel ready!

We woke up the next morning hopeful and nervous. I had one test left in my luggage. We got online with the lab, which walked us through the Antigen test. After fifteen minutes, the results came back negative, so I knew we had only a twenty-four-hour window to get out the country. Anxiety ran through me as I scrambled to get our luggage, passports, test results, and new flights all in place to get us out.

After we rushed to the airport, we got in line. But we weren't out of the woods yet. When we reached the ticket agent, he took a look at our documentation and said, "Your test results are valid, but your daughter's are not."

What?!

I questioned the agent as we had used this online lab to get us into Aruba. He replied they had just changed the rules. "You have to get tested by an Aruban lab, not an online lab."

I pleaded with him, telling him the flight left in two hours, adding that no one told me of this change, asking how we could possibly make the flight in time. Unmoved, he directed us to go down the street to a lab at a hotel to get Ashley retested.

Ashley and I picked up our things and started running. When we arrived at the lab, the man at the desk said they were too busy to do the fifteen-minute test and that we had no choice but to wait one hour for her results. He instructed us to go back to the airport and that her results would be emailed to us.

I had to sit with my adrenaline pulsing through my veins waiting for one hour for her test results. I was clearly anxious, and my daughter could see it. I imagined us stuck without a hotel in a foreign country. We would have to test again tomorrow. The what ifs came flooding into my brain. *What if I tested positive tomorrow?* I had to sit with the uncomfortable feelings of anxiety and fear, which had pulled up a chair up to my table.

I view these feelings like *Sesame Street* monsters. Fear is a hairy, purple monster with crazy-looking eyes. Anxiety is a hot pink monster with wild, stringy hair who can't sit still. They both sit at my table, waiting to see how I will deal with them and their insanity. I see them both and say to myself, *Oh, it's you two again. I see you. I don't like when you come to my table. You both look silly.*

Since being alcohol-free for two years now, I stared at those feelings head-on and saw them for what they were—just feelings that will eventually pass. Silly monsters that appear from time to time. I had no choice but to sit with them, *feel* them, as I waited for

Ashley's test results. I took several deep breaths and began repeating one word to myself . . . *trust.* I had to trust it would all work out. I had to let it go; I had no control.

It was now an hour and ten minutes later—*still* no results in my email. I must have refreshed my email three hundred times. I went back up to the ticket agent, ramping up the intensity: "We may miss the flight. I paid your lab, and I have no test results. It's been over an hour, what do I *do*?"

"We have nothing to do with the lab," he replied. "You have to go back to the lab and get the results to get on this flight."

In the pouring rain, I ran back down the street to the lab. Out of breath, I opened the door to the lab and the gentlemen at the desk looked up at me saying, "I just sent your daughter's results to your email."

"What are the results?" I asked shakily, my words trembling as I tried to catch my breath.

He replied, "Negative."

I took a big exhale and just started running back toward the airport.

Now the flight was one hour away from leaving. We still had to get through customs and several checkpoints to get to our gate. My body was still shaking with anticipation, not sure if we would make it to the gate on time. Each checkpoint was one more test of patience. Then, like a beacon of light, I saw the words "Philadelphia Flight 504: *On Time*." We had made it to our gate.

When we got home, I called my mom and my mother-in-law to fill them in on our ordeal. After hearing about the debacle, both both of them said, "I bet you had a drink after all that!"

I simply replied, "Nope."

I had sat with all the anxiety, body trembling, praying for negative test results, uncertainty pounding against my chest and then, just like that, the monsters left my table.

The "F*ck-It Moments" are just that . . . moments. Moments to grow comfortable with the uncomfortable, acknowledging that this too shall pass. My daughter saw all my fear, uncertainty, and anxiety. I'd much rather she see her role model face uncertainty and forge through it rather than me washing it all down with a drink to cope with it. I couldn't hide my fear, nor should I. My kids deserve to see a mother who doesn't pad herself at every challenge in life: They see someone who might not handle every situation perfectly but in the best way she can—messy yet beautiful. They need to see that there will be times in life that can rock even their biggest role model but that she can make it through without alcohol. I fully recognize that sometimes our biggest challenges don't resolve that quickly, but the hard, sharp, edgy feelings do soften over time.

A few weeks after our return from Aruba, I received a call from Susie, one of the girls in my Sober Sis group, who was hitting her own "F*ck-It Moment." As a retired medical device salesperson and mother to four kids, she and I had bonded over both being in the medical sales industry. Even though it had been a year and half of Susie not even taking one sip of alcohol, now she was on the brink of throwing in the towel and getting a drink. She was tired, her new dosage for her depression medication was off, her therapist was on vacation, and she had hit a breaking point. She had been fighting with her son, who always was a challenge for her, and this time she could not take it anymore. I listened to her vent, validated her raw emotions, and then said, "What do you think alcohol would provide for you?"

"I know, I know," she replied, "but I just don't want to feel any of this anymore."

I continued: "I understand, you want to check out. But play it forward. You will wake up tomorrow to these same issues that alcohol will not make go away . . . and you will feel like crap on top of it."

There was a long pause and then Susie said, "I know."

I knew she knew in her heart the truth, but she was circling the pitcher plant after a year and half of walking away from it. I wanted her to think long and hard about her choice to go back into the trap, so I said, "What would you tell your daughter to do if she was coming to you with these same issues? Would you tell her to go get a drink, or would you tell her to take a walk, maybe a long hot bath, or journal how she was feeling?"

Susie paused, took a deep breath, and then responded, "You're right, I would not tell her to escape in a drink."

"Good," I replied, "Now go model it for her."

Susie called me the next day to thank me. She was *so* grateful she did not fall back into the pitcher plant's deception.

"You did this," I told her. "You made the right choice; you rescued yourself. I just walked alongside you and held your hand."

Moving Forward

The alcohol-free journey may look like an impossible mountain to conquer, but we don't hike up the precipice, we hike *through* it together. What was essential for me was staying in a community of women who got it even a year and half later, when we all thought we were out of alcohol's prison but discovered we were still vulnerable to alcohol's abusive ways. Even though we were not thinking about alcohol nearly as much as we did at the beginning of our journey, it did not mean we were not still susceptible to it. By keeping the conversation going on the illusions of what we thought alcohol provided, we were further ingraining the truths about alcohol into our minds.

I could see the alcohol trap I fell into and worked so hard to escape. Drinking amnesia is a real thing! Staying connected to women who wanted to remain on this path of being alcohol-free forever was key in my success.

Choosing not to drink is the greatest act of self-love imaginable . . . facing and understanding your triggers, showing up clear-minded, fighting the uncomfortable over choosing to escape. Getting comfortable with the uncomfortable and returning to your true self is challenging. It threatens who we have been told we are for years by society, our families, and ourselves. Alcohol separates us from ourselves. But she is who we must look at with admiration for the strength, tenacity, and perseverance to choose yourself over dodging the pain. It is much easier to check out or go on autopilot, but we can choose to show up for ourselves with grace and patience even when she is exhausted and tired. You just need rest, not a drink. At the core of each of us is love and lots of feelings teaching us, if we are open to it, how to return to love. It isn't easy.

Now I stop and pause, seeing my old self and the old ways of reacting to challenges. This is where I choose again. I acknowledge the past habitual coping mechanisms, as I was doing the best I could at the time, and now choose differently. It has taken loads of work with my therapist, accountability with my Sober Sis group, books, and podcasts to get to a place to see the old me and choose the true me. I don't always do it; it's so easy to just respond the old way I have for over forty years. But just like the sober-curious journey is not perfect nor linear, neither is shifting into a new you. It takes time, practice, and a repetitive letting go of the old ways.

The most rewarding part of the journey is how your mind and body truly change.

The Alcohol-Free Wins Continue in Year Two

I went out to dinner to celebrate my second year of sobriety with some family members. I ordered a Heineken 0.0 with my meal.

When the waiter arrived, he placed the beer on the table with the label facing away from me. I began to sip on my nonalcoholic beer. After a few minutes, I felt funny. My face felt flushed. My body was sending off warning signs that something wasn't right. I turned the bottle around and saw it was a regular Heineken with alcohol. I was proud of my body alerting me to the presence of the alcohol. I was so in tune and aligned with my body that even a few sips set off my internal alarm system!

I waived down the waiter, who apologetically replaced my beer.

Celebrating wins even two years after being alcohol-free continued in my alcohol-free journey. I was given shocking news at the doctor's that I would have to have surgery for a fall from which I had not recovered properly. My mind raced with work and family obligations on the calendar. I would have to be out of work for six weeks. It was jarring and completely unexpected, to say the least.

I understandably had several emotions and reactions to the news. In the past my mind would have said, *We definitely deserve a drink!* Now it said, *We need to go for a walk to process all this*!

Can you say *win*?! My first thought was a healthy solution. My brain had rewired itself: it *can* happen ladies, it just takes time.

As I reflect on 2020 and 2021, it was the time I went against the grain. I took the leap of faith to listen to my inner knowing that alcohol was not serving me: it was making me sick. It was uncomfortable and hard, as everyone around me was leaning into alcohol to get through the pandemic. Going against what appears to be normal is always awkward, hard, and sometimes feels impossible. But by not joining the masses and choosing not to drink, I learned for the first time in my life how to meet my needs first and not others'. I found the courage within to find my voice and stand up for what I believed in. Courage does not come from a can but from choosing yourself *first*, listening to that deep inner knowing who is guiding you in the right direction.

The first year of being alcohol-free was like waking up to everything I had been asleep to for years. It was the year of the dense fog lifting, awakening, yielding to the present, and clearly seeing who I wanted to be.

At the beginning of being alcohol-free, I thought, *Am I going to have to think about being alcohol-free every day*? Now, at over two years alcohol-free, I don't think about alcohol much, but every day I do reflect on how I can reconnect with my true self. The very thing (alcohol) that brought us to our knees is also the very thing that will rescue you. I have become my own refuge.

I had been awakened to my one wild and precious life.

The freedom I gained from my journey has helped keep me alcohol-free to this day. Every hard turn in life would now be an opportunity to slow down, hit pause, and explore the wilderness of what it was there to teach me. It isn't always easy, but each challenge is an opportunity to grow into the best version of myself. Living in "AF Awakened Freedom,"[2] coined by Jenn Kautsch, allows us to live authentically free and wholeheartedly. No longer do I want to use a depressant to celebrate or just *rest*.

Looking back, I'm certain my inner knowing was always pointing me toward freedom, but I relied on external opinions and approvals as my compass for guidance. My role models are no longer supermodels but women who are authentically and vulnerably themselves, fearlessly pronouncing their truths through their seminars, podcasts, and books, and who are quoted in this book: Brené Brown, Glennon and Amanda Doyle, Jolene Park, Laura McKowen, Jenn Kautsch, and Holly Whitaker. By becoming free of the chains of alcohol, your new freedom allows you to dictate when and how you have fun, when and how you rest. No more back and forth of can I, should I, or shouldn't I drink. Your newfound freedom looks much like this:

- Freedom from how much is too much
- Freedom from the decision fatigue on whether or not to moderate
- Freedom from hangovers
- Freedom from the gray fog that covered your lens each day
- Freedom from shame and guilt
- Freedom from drama
- Freedom from external validations
- Freedom from not having enough time to more time
- Freedom that alcohol is no longer in control of you
- Freedom from everything you thought alcohol provided when it did not
- Freedom from the façade, the show
- Freedom from all the lies we believed

Most importantly, you're free to be ***you***.

Being liberated from the pitcher plant and its lure is the truest freedom. Free from trying to find rest and peace in alcohol when it only adds stress and anxiety. I was finally free from the gray area drinking merry-go-round, the "detox just to retox" loop,[3] and the never-ending spin cycle. No longer am I a divided woman with divided thoughts but rather a woman who has stepped into trusting herself above all else. Like the wind, uncertain of which way it will blow, relying on external validation leaves you always relying on the uncertainty outside of yourself.

I was free from serving as the "number-two rescuer" as well. When your role for over forty years was to be the fixer, rescuer, and in control, just sitting with someone's pain can be very challenging. When we learn to do this with ourselves, we can do this for others. We abandon ourselves when we let worry, fear, and anxiety take over our nervous system. When we can sit with ourselves in the good and the bad, we are showing up for ourselves. This is not always easy. I am still learning to hold space for those in my life who need to be heard and validated, not rescued or fixed. I am learning to hold space to expand my capacity to sit with a friend's vast pain and not try to resolve it. As hard as this is, the true beauty is allowing that capacity to unfold into her own transformation that she finds within herself.

Finding this transformation allows us to take back our voices of being real, vulnerable, and authentic women who can talk about this highly addictive drug and how we learned through being alcohol-free to be empowered and liberated from the bondage of alcohol. The more real we are with one another, the less the stigma around our hidden secret with alcohol becomes. The truth about our secrets with alcohol connects us and releases us from the chains of gray area drinking.

The Truth: The truth is showing up for yourself, putting yourself first, choosing to stay away from a substance that only takes—not gives—day in and day out is vital because no one else will do it for you. It is your empowered choice, and yours alone. You are the greatest gift to yourself. Once I learned how to fill these spaces with loving myself, I no longer needed a substance, thing, or person to fill them. Now the connection with myself is firm and deep-rooted; I know nothing, not even alcohol, would come between us again. I get to get up each day and rescue her from who she used to be and how God intended her to live. My refuge lives deep within me; *nothing* and *no one* can take it from me. It is a safe place, like the bay, a place where the storms of life may surround me but where I am anchored in the unconditional love of who I am now.

Did You Know?

According to the 2014 World Cancer Report (WCR), "No amount of alcohol is safe."[4]

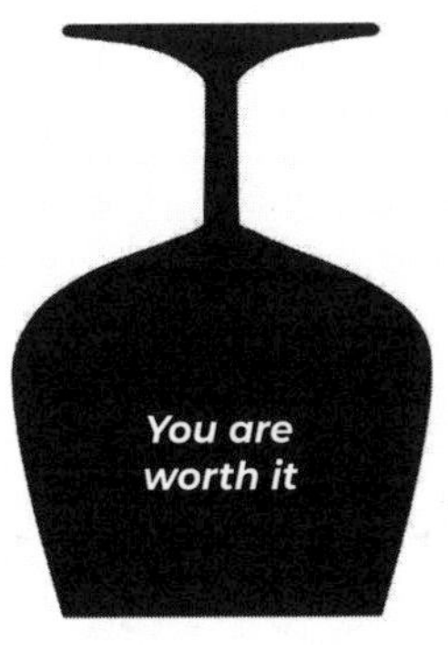

CHAPTER EIGHT

THE TRUTH OF WHO YOU ARE

It was time for my weekly call with Cari, my transformational life coach, who would guide me through my past traumas with all the wisdom and insight of all my former therapists combined. After listening to another one of my past stories, she looked at me inquisitively over Zoom and asked, "Who is Meg?"

I just stared blankly at the screen, digging deep within for the answer. I began to ponder: *Who am I*?

Usually, the first thing that comes to mind is the roles we fulfill as mother, wife, sister, career professional, caretaker—all the roles of who I was or should be, but now that I could see through these so-called roles, I got very still and quiet, leaning into that deep space within, searching for the answer. Then the little girl within arose, beaming her bright, guiding light, and I replied, "She is a loving and compassionate person who cares deeply about people."

Cari began nodding her head on the screen in agreement then said these four words I will never forget: "And that is *enough*."

The truth is: *You* are enough.

No one had ever said these words to me before. All my life, I was chasing a belief of who I thought I had to be to prove my enough-ness, my worth. For most of my life, I was doing and escaping, distracting from the limited beliefs bestowed upon me when the truest, most right answer was right there all along inside of me. I could finally *exhale*. Over forty years of exhaustion now poured with my tears into a release I had never felt before.

Our true self is like a rare gem who has been buried deep within the earth's layers. We see her glimpses of her bright light, glowing and illuminating the pathway to the truth in our lives. It is our choice to tune into that light, our inner knowing.

As we work through each layer of our conditioning, unearthing her, we can see she has always been our guiding light, shining her truth up through us our entire lives. When we cherish her as the dazzling, rare gem that she is, we can see that *she is enough*. The fear of not doing enough, of not being enough, the fear of failure: Your old, conditioned beliefs are burned to the ground by her blazing, brilliant, bright light. I now trust my inner knowing, listening, and letting her brilliance guide me.

Burning down these societal, familial, and cultural beliefs is paramount to this transformation. It requires taking the time to get quiet and tune into what the little girl within you is saying because the truth lives within *you*. You are already listening to her: She is the very thing that brought you here to this book, guiding you on your path.

Stay true to you, no matter what society tells you. Change is hard. But vulnerability, authenticity, and connection are the path to courage to transform into the best version of you. It takes time and it is not linear. There are bumps, twists, turns, and challenges along the way. They are there for a purpose: to guide you, to teach you. To push you along your own unique path.

It takes alcohol being removed for an extended period of time (or forever) to tap back into your inner knowing. Your inner knowing has always been there but has been dimmed by the billion-dollar alcohol industry and our alcohol-centric society. Once you are alcohol-free, you learn how to build your confidence again based on this inner knowing. She knows she is right. She knows what she wants. Her voice is no longer silenced. She starts to come alive with opinions and truths. She is no longer indecisive. She is grounded in who she is.

She is waiting for you to rescue her. She is longing for her voice to sing from the rooftops again like she did when she was a little girl. When she steps into her worth, she finds her voice. She is strong and she is enough. Her "perfect" is redefined by being good enough for *herself*. She no longer needs validation from the external world. She now gives that to herself, feeding her inner knowing.

I continue to shift away from perfectionism. I say "continue" because it's an undoing process of over forty years of a coping mechanism. One that *didn't* work.

When we are trying to control everything, we are not trusting ourselves. We used alcohol to release us from this feeling of having to control everything. Alcohol may numb you initially for a few minutes (remember, alcohol's buzz only lasts twenty minutes), but overall, it disconnects you from yourself, not allowing you to be still and feel your inner knowing. When we cannot connect to ourselves, we cannot trust ourselves.

Trusting my own judgment again was like a snake shedding her old skin. A snake sheds its skin four to twelve times a year. The process is a necessary one to fully enter into the best version of yourself. There is no shame in the old skin that sheds off. A snake's skin comes off all in one piece, which allows you to see the outline of her old body, her old life. Her old skin, her past which made her who she is today, is not a reflection of shame or guilt but rather an old form of herself that was constricted by society, trauma, or familial or cultural beliefs.

This repetitive shedding is how we outgrow and heal our past. I could see now that some of the roots of my shame were the unrealistic expectations placed on me when I was younger. Because I could not fulfill these expectations, like taking care of my brother and sister through my parents' divorce, it catapulted me into feeling shameful for not being enough or doing enough. Eventually, with Cari's guidance, I learned to forgive myself for shaming myself and judging myself as not enough. And I forgave myself for the misunderstanding, misbelief, and judgment I placed upon myself of always thinking I needed to just do more to make up for my perceived shortcomings. I was coping the best way I knew how.

The Machine

So when did we lose ourselves? We have already discussed the old, programmed beliefs, roles, expectations, and messages we get from a young age from our families, culture, and society. Then you add in the "machine" of productivity culture, which tells us that if we are not hustling and grinding, all while being perfectly successful at it, then we are not enough.

In Martha Beck's book *The Way of Integrity*, she writes, "Anything you do solely to influence others, rather than to express your true nature, is a hustle."[1]

We live in a culture where our value is placed on our hustle. The constant messages that you are worth what is in your bank account or how many followers you have on social media or by participating in diets/challenges/programs create a huge burden on our shoulders—coupled with the fact that if we don't do it perfectly, we are a failure.

We measure ourselves in absolutes and perfectionism. For example, if you join a fitness challenge and it says to work out sixty minutes a day, we think we are a failure for only working out forty-five or fifty minutes. I have been in several challenges where my accountability partner felt like a failure for not hitting these absolute measures put into place by the challenge instead of seeing the great progress she had made simply by participating. The machine is wearing us down to paper-thin versions of ourselves, where there is no room for imperfection.

We are drawn to these limited-time challenges because we want quick fixes to improve ourselves. We are an instant gratification society that expects perfection within thirty days or less. I can tell you it took me at least a hundred days or more to really feel like I was on the other side of alcohol. I couldn't even see how gray my life was until I had removed it for an extended period of time. I am not pointing fingers; I too have joined these programs and challenges. The 21-Day Reset is why I am here, but we have to give ourselves more grace and time for true change. If I have learned one thing on this journey, it is that everyone's alcohol-free journey looks different and has taken various amounts of time. It isn't cookie cutter in a shiny, little box of thirty days or less.

We have been taught since we were little girls to look outside of ourselves for what we should desire rather than listening to what we truly desire. Getting conflicting messages throughout our lives on how we should look, behave, and think from our culture, society, and even our own family leads us to not trust ourselves. We listen to the consensus, the masses, the outside voices of what we *should* do or what *everyone else* is doing rather than our clear, definitive, most true inner voice.

We find it hard to relax because we've been conditioned to judge ourselves by what we are doing externally to prove ourselves or to be worthy or even *valued*—rather than coming from a space of knowing our worth and that we *deserve* to just rest. Many of us, sadly, don't even know what rest looks like (refer back to *Finding Your Fun Self* in chapter 4). The ever-spinning vortex of the machine has robbed us of knowing our own needs and joys.

Even as we grow and evolve, we fear we will be a fraud if we falter, but isn't it in the so-called failures and sidesteps that we climb to the next level of becoming our true selves?

This is why the inner work never *ends.*

It's letting go of the what ifs, releasing ourselves of the perfect absolutes, and finding our truths in what is true right now. Our feelings and coping mechanisms are protectors who have helped protect us through much of our lives. When we view them as such, we can let go of the shame. Our protectors are there to guide us back to integrity. This allows for more space for radical self-love and acceptance.

Our mental health is something we have to work on daily, just like our physical health. We don't just wake up in tip-top shape; we have to commit to work on it every day. The same is true for our mental health.

Healing the Little Girl Within

As I was learning, with Cari's guidance, how to tune into my inner knowing, it was time to heal the little girl who was so wounded by my past sexual assaults. We got online for our weekly call and Cari had me close my eyes and take several deep breaths. Then she had me visualize being back behind the bush where I was attacked.

I felt as though I was hovering over my body, lying there paralyzed by someone taking complete control over me and my body. Tears welled up in my eyes as I could feel the fear, the terror, and the uncertainty of potentially being raped rise back up in my body even though it had been twenty years ago.

In her soothing manner, Cari then said, "Now I want you to place your adult-self next to her, with all her fears, all the feelings of loss of control, and uncertainty. Just breathe, let her know you are there, we got this, just be there with her. What do you want to say to her in that moment?"

Immediately, I was no longer hovering over myself but rather down on the ground, immersed in the leaves with her. I wrapped myself around her on the ground in an enveloping, warm, safe hug. I whispered to my hurting little girl, *I am here for you, you are not alone. This is not right; this is not your fault. We will be okay*. Tears were now pouring out of my soul, relinquishing the pain, the hurt, and the fear that had lived in my body for over twenty years.

After I took a few deep breaths, Cari had me visualize myself after my date rape. The feelings of unworthiness, of utter violation, rushed back into my body. The shame was so encompassing that I felt like I could not tell anyone. It was my shameful secret where, again, it felt like it was my fault because I had drunk too much. I was lying in my bed, curled up into a ball, where I stayed for days after this violation. I had no desire to participate in life. I felt like damaged goods.

Then Cari had me envision my adult-self crawling into bed with her, spooning her, wrapping myself around the little girl who felt so unworthy, telling her, "This doesn't define you. This is not your fault; this was a complete violation. You will find someone who will love you unconditionally."

Cari responded, "And that is the truth; breathe that in. Let her receive that because *she is still in you*. That girl who wondered, 'Who will ever love me; will I be loved again?' You are safe; you are okay."

Suddenly the darkness gave way to light, where my inner gem's warm, golden light, like that of a soft glowing candle, wrapped itself around me in unconditional, nonjudgmental, pure love where true healing took place.

Cari went on to say, "The key is when you feel the old programming of distraction, of achievement, and of unworthiness pop up, do not look at it with judgment, but rather say 'Of course this is coming up, of course you are responding this way,' because that is a trauma response. View it with compassion and understanding."

I cannot take away what happened to me, but I had shifted the energy around it. I had rescued and healed my own self with Cari's loving guidance.

This is where a somatic therapist or life coach is key. We need to normalize mental health and trauma support. Most of us are suffering from something. These trained experts can help you navigate through these hard feelings. You are not supposed to do this alone. A sobriety support group can also help you see you are not alone. If hiring a therapist or joining a support group is not an option for you, there are many free podcasts and online resources that can help you move through these emotions as well.

Tapping Back into Your Inner Knowing

We are not trained to go inward. Again, we are conditioned to look outside ourselves for our worth, value, and approval. By choosing to become alcohol-free, it forced me to go inward.

Meditation was not something I had ever done before. When I first started meditating in my alcohol-free journey, I did only guided meditations. They are a great place to start. One of the best guided meditations I have listened to on this journey is Sarah Blondin's *Discovering Your Intrinsic Self* on Insight Timer. Insight Timer is a free app with thousands of guided meditations.

Slowing down and giving your mind time to process all the changes on your alcohol-free journey is vital. The same feeling I would get from the first glass of wine (the twenty-minute decompression period) I found I could get from meditation. My clenched jaw, stiff back, and endless to-do list would melt away with each deep breath. Wine did not cure my stress; if anything, it just pushed it off to be dealt with later, which only compounded it. Meditation gives me true stress relief, but initially I was not doing it every day.

Later in my journey, I joined a program Cari created called "Shift into Alignment." During her program, she had us meditate every day for fifteen minutes, in total silence. No voices or music to distract our minds.

At first, I asked myself, *Will I have the time to do this every day? Can I sit in total silence with my monkey mind?*

Every day, I sat on a little blue pillow and lit a candle in front of me to help me to stay present. Each day, more of my inner knowing would show up, guiding me, revealing to me more of my true self.

Daily meditation has been life changing for me. Tuning into myself was something I had never explored before . . . that is, until I started working with Cari. I am now able to drop into my inner knowing on a daily basis and listen to what my mind, body, and spirit are telling me. It has allowed me to regulate my nervous system by grounding my anxiety.

There is no wrong or right way to meditate. Find a quiet place where you can sit, relax, and open up to what your inner knowing is trying to tell you. Some days I just feel peace; other days, my monkey mind races with thoughts. Don't judge your meditations, just let them be. To ground myself even further, I meditate while taking long warm baths. Taking baths early on in my alcohol-free journey were paramount to unwinding from a stressful day. Today, baths with meditation represent a place of feeling held and grounded with an overwhelming sense of peacefulness. Discovering this deep peace within allows me to let go of the perfectionism, the chronic people pleasing, and the need to always strive, push, and do more.

My meditations have been evolving on my journey. I recently came up with an idea to do a "I AM" meditation. For fifteen minutes, I tell myself only positive words about what I am relative to my mind, body, and spirit. Try it! You will stand a little taller afterward, feeling your worth, knowing God made you perfectly as you are. We can give ourselves the confidence we need, not in an egotistical way but rather from a place of truly knowing our worth.

Now my daily meditations are more like prayers. I ask God to allow me to be a conduit for His will. I let go of all the need to control and hand it all over to Him. I ask Him to use me as His vessel for the truth to set women free. This two-way prayer was inspired by Elizabeth Gilbert, author of *Eat, Pray, Love*, who shared this morning ritual on Glennon Doyle's podcast, *We Can Do Hard Things*, episode 95.[2]

Here is an example of my morning prayer:

> Dear God,
>
> What is your will for me today? Let me be a conduit for your will. Inspire my writing for me today. I ask for your

> wise words to free women of the limiting beliefs that are bestowed upon them. May my creativity come from you. I release all need to control and worry about how this book will launch into the world. I hand this book over to you. May it be in service to you and to so many women who need to hear the truth not only about alcohol but also about their worthiness.

In my heart and my mind, I hear in response,

> Dear Precious One,
>
> I hear your heart. I see your truth. I am always with you. I see the fear in your eyes from time to time. You are not one with this world that makes you believe you need to market, push, or force your creativity upon it. Trust in me. I have always held you and always will. No one, nothing can stop my will to help these women. Let go of the limiting beliefs you place upon yourself as well. Know I am always here guiding you. Stand tall in the truth we have written together.

I had finally come to a place in my journey where I could see my one true self and trust my inner knowing, no matter what or who told me otherwise. I can see I am a reflection of God. It means seeing there is so much more to this one precious life than choosing a substance that takes versus gives. I had shifted to my heart—to my one *true* self—where all my power fully lives. Each time life's storms brewed up and cast their shadow down upon me, I realized how my reaction to these blows were just as important. In the beginning, my reactions were just as intense as the storm then . . . over time, something beautiful was given to me. Like a gift, I began to unwrap and learn who I was and why my reactions were the way they were.

This gift, once opened, gave me more peace and less drama in my life. It continues to give by allowing me to be more present and less reactive. Laura McKowen brilliantly named her book *We Are the Luckiest* because we *are* the luckiest to have been given this journey of self-discovery when we choose to become alcohol-free.

The feelings still arise, and life continues to be challenging, but I am so grateful to have reconnected with myself, my inner knowing. I am still learning; the inner work is never done, it isn't perfect, but neither am I.

CONCLUSION

In the story *The Little Engine That Could,* the toys and food all need to be taken over the mountain after their engine breaks down. They ask three engines who are passing by for help, all of whom reply they are too good or too fancy to pull just food and toys over the mountain. Then the blue engine comes along, unsure of her capabilities and worth, but she decides to help anyway.

She pushes herself, saying, *I think can—I think I can—I think I can*, pushing, striving, and hustling until she tugs the toys and food over the mountain.

We are programmed from an early age to push and power our engines, chugging through the mountains life puts in our paths. Looking back on the tracks of my life, my engine didn't stop hustling and grinding—I didn't get still for a very long time—until I stopped drinking.

What my engine really needed was to rest, to get still, to pause, and to actually *listen* to her inner knowing. God is the engineer of my engine now as I have relinquished the need for the *illusion* of control. I no longer look outside myself for validation. My engine still gets tired, life doesn't stop, but I know now how to care for my engine and listen to her guiding me around the bends of life. I listen to what brings her joy, flow, and purpose. Without this addictive substance in the way, my engine could finally rest, knowing she is enough, just as God made her.

NOTE FROM THE AUTHOR

Can we take a minute, ladies? Can we slow down to celebrate our accomplishments and wins? As I was finishing this book, I was overwhelmed with the next steps of birthing it into the world. My sister reminded me, "Can we just take a minute and celebrate that you got sober during a pandemic and wrote a book?"

Like so much of what my sister says to me, she stops me in my tracks. Tears start to stream out of my eyes. She is right. I hadn't even celebrated the fact that I finished writing this book. A book that has cathartically taken me on a journey of self-discovery and self-healing. It's taken me almost two years to write, yet I haven't even realized that I had not allowed myself a minute of celebrating this creation.

Take a minute to celebrate your wins, no matter how big or small they may be. It's important to honor your pivot, your transformation, your new habits, your accomplishments, and your choice to stay alcohol-free for another day. It's here in the wins that we can reflect and see the true you, the most beautiful version of you who appears. Celebrate *that*, Sister!

Launching this book into the Universe felt daunting at first. I was no expert in social media, nor do I have a business platform related to this book. I am just an ordinary mom who felt her truth and story needed to be heard to flip the script on the mommy wine culture. My hope is that you can see the imperfection of my journey when I debated slipping back into my old ways. I challenge the big alcohol industry for the trap they have created—in particular, for making women believe they deserve a glass of wine rather than rest, radical self-love, and appreciation for all the contributions they pour into their homes and into the world.

As I wrap this book up, it's Easter and I can't help but reflect on rebirth. Nature provides us with so many examples of shedding the old (like the snake's skin I mentioned earlier) and blooming with the new. We are taught in our culture to just persevere through it, but nature's consistent examples of rebirth tell us otherwise. I hear from women all the time about all the shame and guilt they carry from their past behaviors. Like a snake sheds her skin, let it go, shed that shit. As my good friend says, "Shame off you!"

> If the pain was deep you will have to let it go many times. Letting go is not a one-time event; it is a habit that requires consistent repetition to become strong.
>
> —Yung Pueblo, Author[1]

TOOLS TO EXPLORE YOUR ALCOHOL-FREE JOURNEY

Connection & Feedback

Think of birds flying in a V formation—one bird flies at the front as the leader, while the other birds follow. Then, when the leader gets tired and falls back, the next bird in line steps up to cut through the wind and lead the group.

This is what Sober Sis, my SoberMinded Sisterhood, was to me. When one of us was down, another would step up with encouragement. Incredible women, all suffering with life's greatest challenges, looking for a way out of the mental mind-f*ck of alcohol. We could see our struggles and wins in each other. We shared our learnings from podcasts, books, and emails, helping lift the other on their path to sobriety. Our daily personal videos on Marco Polo were, in essence, pushing us along on the alcohol-free journey. We bonded over shared trials and tribulations when alcohol took us down.

We realized we were not crazy, that this mental mind game was going on in all of our heads. We realized we were not alone. When one of us would isolate or not be on Marco Polo for a few days or weeks, we would call out their name on our video posts, asking, "Where are you; how are you doing? No judgment, just come back to us and tell us what is happening on your journey." We just kept showing up for each other. Time and time again.

With no judgment, no failure, and only unconditional love and support, it created a safe space where we could show up messy, vulnerable, and authentically ourselves. By figuring it out at our own pace, in our own way, each of us was successful in this alcohol-free exploration by drinking less or being totally alcohol-free. *None* of us could look at alcohol the same again. It was like a divine group of women put together by the grace of God; when life brought on a challenge, someone in the group would say, "I have walked that pain. I know that journey. You are not alone. I am here to help you; I will walk with you through this . . . and *not* with a drink in hand!" It was a safe place where we each lifted each other up. Reminding each other of the tools we had learned in our program and how to use them successfully.

Much like female elephants who protect each other, this group of women showed up for one another in our moments of weakness and strength. Female elephants surround one of their own mommas when she is giving birth. They gather around her in a circle, with their backs to her, essentially on the lookout, protecting her from danger. As the momma elephant begins her labor and birthing process, her protective tribe stirs up dust with their feet to protect and hide the momma and her baby.

This is what my Sober Sis group was to me. A tight-knit circle of friends who were protecting, watching, looking out for, and birthing my sobriety.

This is key to staying alcohol-free. Walking the path with others in a support group who can relate and understand your challenges along the way. It is important to find a group that mirrors what your struggle looks like. There are so many different types of sober support groups out there. Join a call; take part in a virtual or in-person meeting—where you see yourself and your relationship with alcohol in the stories of others—that is where you belong.

As Jenn Kautsch of Sober Sis says, "Connection is the secret sauce to our program."[1] Research shows that we heal better in community. When we are overwhelmed and exhausted, we need to know we are not alone. Being part of a community of women who struggle with similar burdens and expectations allows us to be seen and say, "That's how I feel." We don't deserve wine; we deserve to be held and heard in community.

Self-Care

In my experience, the most critical tool in the alcohol-free journey is self-care. If you are choosing to not drink, you are prioritizing yourself. It is paramount to put yourself first. When you put yourself first, you will no longer need a substance to "take care of you."

Throughout this transformation, connection to myself was key. I had to learn to take care of myself first. Choosing and putting yourself first is not selfish. It is a daily gift that we give ourselves!

In the past, I was trying to find my self-care and hopes for an answer at the bottom of a bottle, neither of which was there. Shifts in your life will occur, but I can promise you there is a clearer, more present, happier, healthier version of you waiting for you to rescue her on the other side.

Self-care can look like spending time in nature, meditation, or in journaling where it allows your mind to process and retrain your thoughts. Grounding yourself in your body and spirit are paramount to shifting into a calmer, more peaceful state of mind. This takes time. Baby steps. Be gentle with yourself. Life will keep throwing you challenges, but returning to self-care will be the way through them.

Getting to know yourself better with the Enneagram is also very insightful. You can find a free Enneagram test online at truity.com.

Movement

Another nonnegotiable for me in my alcohol-free journey is movement. Movement is medicine. This time is my time to nourish my body. The endorphins that are released energize me for the day. Sometimes these workout sessions are a release of anger and frustration. Sometimes they are a gentle walk with a good podcast. Regardless, it is time well spent in becoming the healthiest version of you.

My road bike saved me on my alcohol-free journey. I love being in nature and flying into a meditative state as I pedal around and around. As I pedal up hills, shifting the gears to make it easier, I realize I am in control of my thoughts and emotions. When life is easy, like sailing down the hills on my bike, I can increase the gear to make it feel a bit harder, feeling more in control. Sometime the bike takes over and a rush of speed comes over my legs as I fly down the bike trail—that same exhilarating feeling of knowing and loving myself. Releasing all the judgment I have bestowed upon myself, a true sense of freedom washes over me. Free of my addiction, free of the alcohol mental mind game, free to be me. These rides fill my cup and runneth over.

Recommended Podcasts

- *We Can Do Hard Things* by Glennon Doyle
- *Unlocking Us* by Brené Brown
- *This Naked Mind* by Annie Grace
- *Take A Break from Drinking* by Rachel Hart
- *Tell Me Something True* by Laura McKowen
- *Editing Our Drinking and Our Lives*
  by Jolene Park and Aidan Donnelly Rowley
- *Quitted* by Holly Whitaker and Emily McDowell

Create a Playlist

Some of the songs on my "I Love Me" playlist include:

- "The Greatest" by Sia
- "Me!" by Taylor Swift
- "I Love Me" by Meghan Trainor
- "Come Alive" by Lauren Daigle
- "Part of Me" by Katy Perry
- "I am Woman" by Emmy Meli
- "We Can Do Hard Things" by Tish Melton and Brandi Carlile
- "Home" by Phillip Phillips
- "Inner Peace" and "Darling" by Beautiful Chorus
- "In the Blood" by John Mayer
- "I Won't Back Down" by Imaginary Future
- "Put Down What You are Carrying" by Trevor Hall and Brett Dannen
- "More Than Enough" by Tubby Love
- "This Is Me" by The Greatest Showman

Keep a Journal

All the changes that occur in sobriety can be overwhelming at times, and this is where writing can be cathartic. It is a way of releasing all the bottled-up feelings surging inside of us. The beauty of journaling is that there are no rules. Color, draw, cuss: just write whatever you feel that day in your journal.

Some of the women in my group had never had a journal before and felt intimated by the journaling process. Here are a few journal prompts that can help those who are not sure how to start:

- How do I feel today?
- What am I grateful for?
- Who am I? . . . (*And that's enough*!)
- How am I protecting my energy?
- What have I learned today in my journey?
- What is my why in wanting to be alcohol-free? What things drove me to drink?
- What wins did I have in my alcohol-free journey today/ this week?
- What lies did I believe about alcohol? What is the truth?
- What is my inner knowing telling me? How will she guide me today?
- What did I learn about myself today in meditation?
- What brings me joy?

Looking back on your growth and change throughout your early sobriety is so rewarding. The journal is also there for the days you can't remember why you wanted to be sober in the first place!

For me, the very first page on the first day of being alcohol-free was how alcohol made me feel—why I wanted to stop drinking and what I wanted in life. I reference back to the first day often. It is my anchor. That page reminds me what this journey has given me when I desperately wanted to change. I knew I was stuck in a cycle that was not adding to my life but only detracting from it. Journaling is a great self-care tool that allows your vulnerability and authenticity to show up for yourself on a daily basis. One I particularly recommend is the *Decidedly Dry Journal* by Jessica Steitzer: See Decidedlydry.com.

Zero-Proof Cocktails

Nonalcoholic beers and zero-proof cocktails helped me surf the crave, especially at the beginning of my journey. For some, this may be a trigger, which I can completely understand. For others, it will be the sole way you ward off the wine witch at 5 p.m. Finding a replacement drink was key for me staying alcohol-free. It allowed me to be part of the group at celebrations. And I even noticed that over time, I did not miss the alcohol. *Shocker*: I didn't miss the gasoline!

There are an abundance of zero-proof, alcohol-free beers and wines now available on the market. It's almost overwhelming. Long gone are the days of just one alcohol-free beer available to us.

Having a plan for your alcohol-free drinks is also key. Think ahead to the situations or places that trigger you to want to drink. At the beach, I packed my own nonalcoholic beers in my backpack to not feel like I was missing out on a cold one at the beach. The best part is when everyone is waking up the next day feeling awful, groggy, and with not much energy, you will be popping out of bed looking forward to having a fun, meaningful day. Plus, you can day drink (alcohol-free, of course) and still go to the gym afterward!

These are some of my favorite alcohol-free drinks:

- Heineken 0.0
- Kalo Hemp-Infused Seltzer
- ZeroProof Ritual Tequila
- Any mocktails made with Seedlip
- Leitz Zero-Point-Five Pinot Noir

Boundaries

Boundaries give you the space to grow and feel safe. Creating hard lines in the sand of what works and what does *not* allows you the time and space to heal your past. Some will not want to acknowledge your boundaries; usually these are the people in your life who don't *have* boundaries. Stating our preferences allows us to stop people pleasing and start showing up for only the things in life that bring us joy.

I found boundaries to be one of the hardest things to put into place initially in my alcohol-free journey. As an empath, it is very easy for me to take on others' problems and feelings. It is hard to separate yourself from others, but it is necessary. It also takes practice.

Sticking to your boundaries is also vital but challenging at times. Boundaries give you back your energy. As you become alcohol-free, you will be tapping into your voice more and will want to express what that little girl within truly wants and feels. Boundaries and/or preferences open up the space and capacity to show up for yourself.

Boundary Boss by Terri Cole is a great read on this subject.

EARLY ENTRIES FROM MY ALCOHOL-FREE JOURNAL

Getting sober is much like moving out of your old house (drinking) and building a brand new (alcohol-free) house with your own hands. You have decided to build a new house, one with stronger interior beams. But moving is a pain—the packing of old habits is cumbersome and time consuming. There are boxes and boxes of your stuff: Stuff you haven't dealt with for years. It feels overwhelming and easier to just stay in your old house.

There are many unknowns in building your new home, like how others will view it, especially when you lived in your old house most of your life. But you decide to embark on this new journey, this new life in your new home, without knowing much other than it is time to make a change. You have outgrown your old home. You begin to understand the old house was no longer serving you.

You start by learning how to pour the foundation of self-care and self-love into the new house. Building your new home takes time. There are days you wonder about going back to your old familiar home. There are unforeseen setbacks with building a new home, but you rest on the new, strong foundation you have built, taking it day by day as you continue to build your new home.

As you begin to unpack your boxes of self-loathing, anger, fear, and loneliness, you see that these boxes no longer fit in your new house. You begin to rewire each floor with love, compassion, and healing that fill the rooms with vivid colors. Your hard work starts to reveal that you alone have built a more secure, brighter, clearer house than your old one. Your new home serves you—it *protects* you—and it is where you return for love, safety, and comfort. You are your new home.

The Grip of Alcohol

The dark grip is so tight—
twisted and tangled with fear, anxiety, and pain
It wraps all around my brain—twisting it into total confusion
The grip wrestles with me back and forth, back and forth
Afraid to let go, I hold onto the lies it whispers to steal my soul
Then all at once my soul screams back to let go
Light appears, clarity arises,
and the grip slowly coils back into the darkness
As a new hold wraps my soul of loving myself once again

New Beginnings

My soul is awake
Awake with truth and light
No longer am I a slave to the lies the world has bestowed upon me
I let go of old patterns, thoughts, behaviors
I welcome new beginnings of peace, love, and hope
I am aware of the deep truths that were asleep
for years within my soul
I allow them to rise to the surface
like a new plant reaching for the light
Giving space and time to grow with pain and excitement
as the changes begin within
Changes emerge all around, giving way to new beginnings

ACKNOWLEDGMENTS

This entire book was created by women for women. I looked to many strong women in my life for guidance when I was learning to trust myself. Many of whom are mentioned in this book and so many more that I have been blessed to call friends. I also want to acknowledge my grandmother whose brave and courageous spirit was with me throughout this book journey. I particularly want to acknowledge Jenn Kautsch, whose Sober Sis programs changed the trajectory of my life. Her mentorship and leadership allowed me to step into the greatest transformation of my life, as she calls it, "AF Awakened Freedom."[1] Jenn, you are transforming and freeing the lives of so many women stuck in gray area drinking. I am eternally grateful for your leadership, guidance, programs, and most of all friendship.

I also want to thank my husband, Paul. Your unwavering love and acceptance of me through all my transformations on this journey was the support and rock that I needed to forge forward. You showed up at every transformation with a heartfelt *I am right here with you, supporting you.* You carried the kids, the house, all the things, so I could create this book and birth it into the world. I am forever grateful for your steadfast love and support. You are and always have been our rock. Thank you for crafting the title, *Intoxicating Lies.*

To my family, in particular, my sister, Abby, who has been my greatest teacher. You were the first person to read the first draft and the first person to encourage me to continue when I doubted myself.

In this challenging world, when I feel like a balloon floating up and away, untethered to the earth, you pull me back down to reality and sanity. I could not do this life without you and your wise words. Even though you are my younger sister, you will always be the "older, wiser sister" to me. I am so incredibly grateful to have you in my life. You are a true healer.

To my mom and my dad who have always fostered my gifts, thank you for your support in allowing me to write my truth. You have truly made me feel heard, loved, and validated—the only thing we need from our parents. I am so grateful to you both for your unconditional love and support on this journey. To Alex, Danielle, Jeff, and Paul's family, thank you for your love and support on this journey too. To Suyin, thank you for your feedback. It means more than you know!

To my Sober Sis tribe, the greatest group of women who empower women. Your vulnerability, courage, and bravery to walk this journey together through all its imperfections allowed for a safe space where we all found the beauty in our messes.

To Suzan, you are my go-to girl and one of the first in our group to tell me I should write a book! Thank you for believing in me! Thank you for your patience while I read my first draft to you on Marco Polo! Your nonjudgmental feedback, love, support, and guidance were a beautiful gift that kept on giving on this book journey.

To my early readers and contributors: Suzan, Lily, Eileen, Isabel, Becky, and Susan, thank you for taking the time to make sure I accurately described our journeys together and for sharing your vulnerable stories! Your feedback was vital in shaping the book. Lily, thank you for mentoring me in my early writing process!

To Suzan, Becky, and Lily, thank you for reading multiple copies of my manuscript. I greatly appreciated all the time you took to give me feedback!

To my transformational life coach Cari Rose, who guided me through every feeling, emotion, and trauma that bubbled to the surface after I removed alcohol. You have been such a gift to my life, allowing me to truly find freedom from everything that was holding me back. You helped me listen to my inner knowing and trust her when the world pushed against her. You were the earth school I so desperately needed. I am forever grateful.

To my Shift into Alignment group of women (Suz, Ab, Sarah, Jess, Jen, and Cari), thank you for walking alongside me in this journey with constant encouragement and support to fulfill my purpose.

Suzanne, thank you for your unwavering support when I wanted to throw in the towel. You helped me see my gifts when the imposter syndrome was trying to take over. Thank you for introducing me to Cari. It has been the greatest gift to walk alongside you in this spiritual journey.

To April, thank you for being my so-called Audible audience and helping me with last minute changes. Walking together on this journey with you has been an honor!

To Ariel Curry, this book would not be here without you. As my content editor, you helped me take my early thoughts and transform them into a heartfelt story. Your belief in my writing and storytelling were paramount to me staying the course. You were my go-to person whenever I wasn't sure of the next step in the book journey. You were always there guiding me. I learned so much from you and I am forever grateful for your guidance, expertise, and support.

To Melinda Martin, who got my vision for the book cover and whose talent designed the most beautiful creation for the bookshelves. You are a such an incredible artist! To Gail Fallen, my copyeditor, whose way with words polished my story and allowed my story to flow with your talented editing. You are the best of the best! Thank you for all your encouragement and patience with me!

To Shane Crabtree, at Clovercroft Publishing, who guided me every step of the way to birth this book into the world.

And last, but not least, to my beautiful children Ashley and Grant, who have witnessed and walked alongside me on my alcohol-free journey. It wasn't always easy, but as you said, Ashley, *It was worth it because I have more patience now*. I will always hold dear to my heart, our discussions on the truths about alcohol and the impacts it can have on your life. You both inspire me every day to be the best version of myself. I love you.

ABOUT THE AUTHOR

MEG GEISEWEITE

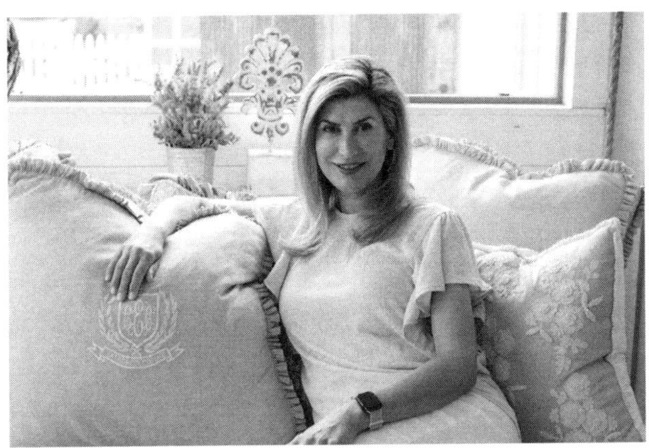

We all want to believe we are in control and have choices in our lives. We want to believe that even the way we let loose and have fun, is just that—*fun*. But slowly, over time, alcohol turns on us, relinquishing our control and leaving us to wonder if it is still any fun.

Meg knew something wasn't right with her relationship with alcohol anymore, but she ignored that small inner voice telling her otherwise. Everyone around her drank just like she did. Never hitting a rock bottom, she struggled silently for years thinking she was alone in her back-and-forth battle with alcohol. When she finally got the courage to tell her therapist she thought she may have a drinking problem, she was told she was thinking about it too much.

These external opinions, combined with no external consequences from her drinking, kept Meg on the "mommy juice" merry-go-round for years.

Meg finally decided to listen to her inner knowing and became sober curious. She found a private, online group of like-minded women from all over the world that felt like she did—trapped by the insidious lies of alcohol. To Meg's surprise, she was not alone;

thousands of women in her Sober Sis group realized that they were trapped in "gray area drinking."

Gray area drinking is a category that exists on the alcohol use disorder spectrum but is rarely discussed. Meg found comfort in knowing she was not alone but was uncertain where her sober-curious journey would take her.

In *Intoxicating Lies*, Meg details the challenges of reclaiming sobriety in our modern culture, a process further complicated by the stress and uncertainty of a global pandemic.

Relatable, riveting, and revealing, *Intoxicating Lies* is both a heartfelt story and a wakeup call for all women, particularly moms trapped in the mommy wine culture. It is the story of how one woman fell not only into alcohol's insidious lies but also the lies our society feeds us to keep women small and silent. *Intoxicating Lies* also shares the stories of the other women in Meg's Sober Sis group whose commonalities created a safe community of ongoing support in her journey. And it's the story of reconnecting to our inner knowing and trusting ourselves to know that, yes, we are enough.

Intoxicating Lies opens the conversation on an epidemic of gray area drinking that is exponentially increasing in women as it flips the script on the alcohol industry.

Connect with Meg

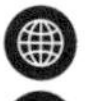 intoxicatinglies.com

 IntoxicatingLiesBook

 Intoxicating Lies: One Woman's Journey to Freedom from Gray Area Drinking

Leave a Review

If you enjoyed *Intoxicating Lies*, will you please leave a review on your platform of choice?

ENDNOTES

Chapter 1

1 Holly Whitaker, *Quit Like a Woman*, (New York, The Dial Press, 2019), 142.

2 American Addiction Centers, "Sexual Assaults on College Campuses Involving Alcohol," updated May 8, 2020, *Alcohol.org*, https://www.alcohol.org/effects/sexual-assault-college-campus/.

Chapter 2

1 Jenn Kautsch, "How to Start an Alcohol-Free Lifestyle," *Sober Sis Blog*, January 10, 2022, https://www.sobersisblog.com/blog-1/how-to-af-living.

2 Ibid.

3 Glennon Doyle, in conversation with Amanda Doyle, June 8, 2021, "Addiction: How Do We Love an Addict and How Does an Addict Love Yourself?" in *We Can Do Hard Things with Glennon Doyle*, podcast, MP3 audio, produced by Candence13, 1:05:37, http://wecandohardthingspodcast.com/.

4 Jolene Park and Aidan Donnelley Rowley, May 29, 2017, "Burnout: Episode 4–Aidan's Stop Story," in *Editing Our Drinking and Our Lives* podcast, MP3 audio, 28:04, https://www.iheart.com/podcast/256-editing-our-drinking-and-o-30942041/episode/episode-4-aidans-stop-story-42573398/.

5 *Merriam-Webster*, s.v. "gray area," https://www.merriam-webster.com/dictionary/gray%20area.

6 Jolene Park, "What Is Gray Area Drinking?" Instagram, February 2, 2022, https://www.instagram.com/p/CZe1dnngy6L/.

7 *Alcohol Research Current Reviews* 39, no. 1 (January 1, 2018), "Drinking Patterns and Their Definitions," National Institute on Alcohol Abuse and Alcoholism, https://arcr.niaaa.nih.gov/binge-drinking-predictors-patterns-and-consequences/drinking-patterns-and-their-definitions.

8 Deborah A. Dawson and Bridget F. Grant, "The 'gray area' of consumption between moderate and risk drinking," *Journal of Studies on Alcohol and Drugs*, vol. 72, 3 (2011): 453-8, doi:10.15288/jsad.2011.72.4537.

9 Jolene Park, "Gray Area Drinking," filmed November 2017 in Denver, Colorado, TED video, 15:05, https://www.ted.com/talks/jolene_park_gray_area_drinking?language=en.

10 US Department of Agriculture and US Department of Health and Human Services, "Dietary Guidelines for Americans, 2020-2025," 9th ed. (December 2020), https://www.dietaryguidelines.gov/resources/2020-2025-dietary-guidelines-online-materials.

11 Ria Health, "Alcohol Use Survey," https://member.riahealth.com/member/alcohol-survey.

12 Jolene Park, "About Gray Area Drinking," Gray Area Drinkers, https://grayareadrinkers.com/about-gray-area-drinking/.

13 Jenn Kautsch, "21-Day Reset!" Sober Sis, https://www.sobersis.com/21-day-challenge.

14 National Institute on Alcohol Abuse and Alcoholism, "Understanding Alcohol Use Disorder," updated April 2021, https://www.niaaa.nih.gov/publications/brochures-and-fact-sheets/understanding-alcohol-use-disorder.

15 Jenn Kautsch (founder, Sober Sis), in phone conversation with author, October 11, 2021.

16 Kari Schwear, "What is Gray Area Drinking?" GrayTonic, https://www.graytonic.com/what-is-gray-area-drinking/.

17 Annie Grace, "Alcohol Only Gives You a 20-Minute High," Instagram, November 13, 2021, https://www.instagram.com/p/CWORzEws59L/.

18 Kristeen Cherney, "Alcohol and Anxiety," Healthline, updated September 26, 2019, https://www.healthline.com/health/alcohol-and-anxiety#:~:text=How%20alcohol%20worsens%20anxiety,an%20entire%20day%20after%20drinking.

Chapter 3

1 Glennon Doyle conversation with Amanda Doyle, in *We Can Do Hard Things*.

2 Health Direct, "Dopamine," last reviewed April 21, 2021, https://www.healthdirect.gov.au/dopamine.

3 William Porter, *Alcohol Explained* (Scotts Valley, CA: CreateSpace Independent Publishing Platform, 2015), 44.

4 Kari Schwear, "You Need This ONE Big Thing, or You May Not Succeed," GrayTonic, https://www.graytonic.com/you-need-this-one-big-thing-or-you-may-not-succeed/.

5 William Porter, speaking during the Sober Sis Quarterly Summit Zoom Call, November 13, 2021.

6 Annie Grace, *This Naked Mind* (New York: Avery, 2018), 52.

7 Grace, *Naked Mind*, 60.

8 Grace, *Naked Mind*, 68.

9 American Cancer Society, "Known and Probable Human Carcinogens," last revised August 14, 2019, https://www.cancer.org/healthy/cancer-causes/general-info/known-and-probable-human-carcinogens.html.

10 National Institute on Alcohol Abuse and Alcoholism, *NIAAA Spectrum* 13, no. 3 (Fall 2021), "As Male and Female Drinking Patterns Become More Similar, Adverse Alcohol Risks for Women Become More Apparent," https://www.spectrum.niaaa.nih.gov/Content/archives/Fall_2021.pdf.

Chapter 4

1 Glennon Doyle, *Carry On, Warrior* (New York: Scribner, 2013), 7.

2 Glennon Doyle, *Untamed* (New York: The Dial Press, 2020), 173.
3 Beatrice Chestnut, *The Complete Enneagram* (Chandler, AZ: She Writes Press, 2013), 19.
4 Brené Brown, "Brené on FFTs," March 20, 2020, in *Unlocking Us with Brené Brown*, podcast, MP3 audio, 37:52, https://open.spotify.com/episode/6UAoHu3VQJNrZcBubo4ABF.
5 Kautsch, "Reset!" Sober Sis.
6 Saundra Dalton-Smith, "The 7 types of rest that every person needs," *Ideas.TED.com*, https://ideas.ted.com/the-7-types-of-rest-that-every-person-needs/.
7 See Cari Rose, Feel the Shift, https://feeltheshift.com/.
8 American Cancer Society, "Human Carcinogens."

Chapter 5

1 Jan Conway, "Sales market share of the United States alcohol industry from 2000 to 2021, by beverage," February 10, 2021, Statista, https://www.statista.com/statistics/233699/market-share-revenue-of-the-us-alcohol-industry-by-beverage/.
2 Kautsch, in phone conversation with author, October 11, 2021.
3 Carrie MacMillan, "Drinking More Than Usual During the COVID-19 Pandemic?" Yale Medicine, June 4, 2020, https://www.yalemedicine.org/news/alcohol-covid.
4 *NIAAA Spectrum*, "Drinking Patterns," Fall 2021.
5 See RAND, "Alcohol Consumption Rises Sharply During Pandemic Shutdown; Heavy Drinking by Women Rises 41%," news release, September 29, 2020, https://www.rand.org/news/press/2020/09/29.html.
6 Batya Swift Yasgur, "Drinking Jumps During Pandemic, Especially in Young Women, WebMD, November 23, 2021, https://www.webmd.com/mental-health/addiction/news/20211123/more-women-drinking-during-pandemic.
7 Brené Brown, "Anxiety, Calm, and Over-/Under-Functioning," April 3, 2020, in *Unlocking Us with Brené Brown*, podcast, MP3 audio, 29:33, https://brenebrown.com/podcast/brene-on-anxiety-calm-over-under-functioning/.
8 Johann Hari, "Everything You Think You Know About Addiction Is Wrong," filmed July 2015 in London, England, TED video, 14:42, https://www.youtube.com/watch?v=PY9DcIMGxMs.
9 Kautsch, "Alcohol-Free Lifestyle," *Sober Sis Blog*.
10 Brené Brown, *Rising Strong: How the Ability to Reset Transforms the Way We Live, Love, Parent, and Lead* (New York: Random House, 2015), 4.
11 Kautsch, "Alcohol-Free Lifestyle," *Sober Sis Blog*.
12 Richie Crowley (@rickieticklez), "7 Predictions for the Non-alcoholic Category in 2021," Medium, https://rickieticklez.medium.com/7-predictions-for-the-non-alcoholic-category-in-2021-f1ccbd3b3a87.

Chapter 6

1 Kautsch, in phone conversation with author.
2 Ibid.

3 William Porter, *Alcohol Explained*, 181.

4 Glennon Doyle, *Get Untamed: The Journal* (New York: Clarkson Potter, 2021), n.p.

5 Tami Simon, in interview with Veronica Valli, January 18, 2022, "A Soberful Life," in *Insights at the Edge*, podcast, MP3 audio, produced by Sounds True, 1:03:03, https://resources.soundstrue.com/podcast/a-soberful-life/.

6 Whitaker, *Quit Like a Woman*, 136.

7 Annie Grace, "Beyond Dry January—Being Alcohol-Free Doesn't Have to End with the Month," accessed June 3, 2022, https://thisnakedmind.com/dry-january-beyond/.

Chapter 7

1 Yung Pueblo (@YungPueblo), Twitter post, November 19, 2019, 1:40 p.m., https://twitter.com/yungpueblo/status/1196890974888382464?lang=en.

2 Ibid.

3 Kautsch, "Alcohol-Free Lifestyle," *Sober Sis Blog*.

4 See Laura A. Stokowski, "No Amount of Alcohol Is Safe," Medscape, April 30, 2014, https://www.medscape.com/viewarticle/824237.

Chapter 8

1 Martha Beck, *The Way of Integrity: Finding the Path to Your True Self* (New York: The Open Field, 2021), 33.

2 Glennon Doyle, in conversation with Elizabeth Gilbert, May 12, 2022, "Why Elizabeth Gilbert Disappeared & What She Came Back to Say," in *We Can Do Hard Things with Glennon Doyle*, podcast, MP3 audio, produced by Candence13, 39:10, https://podcasts.google.com/feed/aHR0cHM6Ly9mZWVkcy5tZWdhcGhvbmUuZm0vd2NkaHQ/episode/YzM2MDE0NmMtM2I1Zi0xMWVjLTkyMmYtNjMzOWRiM2E2MGYx.

Note from the Author

1 Yung Pueblo (@yung_pueblo), "Letting go is not a one-time event . . ." Instagram, March 5, 2022, https://www.instagram.com/p/Caueis8u6NT/.

Tools to Explore Your Alcohol-Free Journey

1 Kautsch, "Alcohol-Free Lifestyle," *Sober Sis Blog*.

Acknowledgments

1 Kautsch, "Reset!" Sober Sis.